Retained Common Duct Stones

Retained Common Duct Stones
Prevention and Treatment

Edited by

Roger W. Motson, MS, FRCS

Consultant Surgeon,
The Colchester Hospitals,
Colchester, Essex,
England

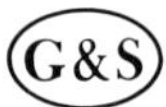

Grune & Stratton
(Harcourt Brace Jovanovich, Publishers)
London   Orlando   San Diego   New York
Toronto   Montreal   Sydney   Tokyo

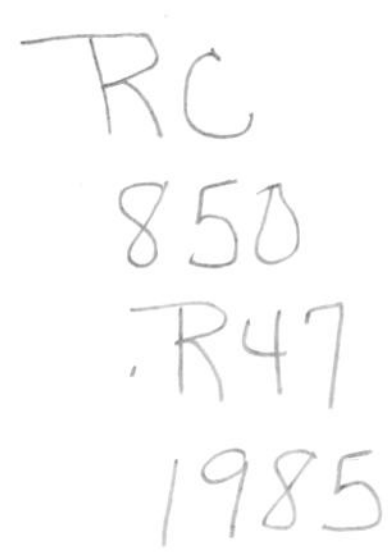

British Library Cataloguing in Publication Data

Retained common duct stones: prevention and treatment.
  1. Gallstones
  I. Motson, Roger W.
  616.3′65   RC850

  ISBN 0–8089–1729–3

Library of Congress Cataloguing in Publication Data

Main entry under title:
Retained common duct stones.
  Includes bibliographies and index.
  1. Calculi, Biliary—Treatment.   2. Calculi, Bilary—Prevention.   3. Calculi,
Biliary—Surgery.   I. Motson, Roger W.   [DNLM: 1. Common Bile Duct Calculi—
prevention and control.   2. Common Bile Duct Calculi—therapy. WI 755 R437]
  RC850.R47   1985   616.3′65   85–5564
  ISBN 0–8089–1729–3

GRUNE & STRATTON, LTD.
24/28 Oval Road
London NW1 7DX

United States edition published by
GRUNE & STRATTON, INC.
Orlando, Florida 32887

International Standard Book Number 0-8089-1729-3
Printed in the United States of America
85 86 87 88   10 9 8 7 6 5 4 3 2 1

List of Contributors

Brian S. Ashby, M Chir, FRCS
Consultant Surgeon, Southend General Hospital, Southend-on-Sea, Essex, England

Adrian R. W. Hatfield, MD, MRCP
Consultant Physician, Department of Gastroenterology, The London Hospital, London, England

Nicolas J. Lygidakis, MD
Associate Professor of Surgery, Department of Surgery, Amsterdam University Medical Centre, Amsterdam, The Netherlands

Richard R. Mason, MRCP, FRCS, FRCR
Consultant Radiologist, The Middlesex Hospital, London, England

Roger W. Motson, MS, FRCS
Consultant Surgeon, The Colchester Hospitals, Colchester, Essex, England; formerly Senior Surgical Registrar, The London Hospital, London, England

Lawrence W. Way, MD
Professor of Surgery, University of California; Chief, Surgical Service, San Francisco V.A. Medical Center, San Francisco, California, U.S.A.

To Jan

Preface

It is less than one hundred years since the common bile duct was first explored for stones. Since then there have been spectacular advances in the safety of cholecystectomy, which is now the most common indication for laparotomy. Advances in surgery for common bile duct stones have been much less spectacular and sadly it remains true that approximately ten percent of patients with common duct stones will not have all their stones removed at the time of cholecystectomy. Operative cholangiography has been available for fifty years but there is still controversy over its efficacy, and the relative merits of supraduodenal versus transduodenal exploration of the bile duct are still debated. However, operative choledochoscopy has now become established and its value is recognized. Despite these efforts at prevention, retained stones continue to occur and are likely to do so for the forseeable future. There have been several developments during the past decade that have completely altered the management of patients with retained stones, and a variety of nonoperative techniques now provide alternatives to a second operation.

I hope that this book will help the reader to keep the incidence of retained stones to a minimum, and assist in choosing the most appropriate technique to use, should a retained stone occur.

I wish to record my thanks to the many surgeons around the world who have responded to my questions in order to clarify the results presented. I am most grateful to them, and to Professor Harding Rains, who first fired my interest in gall-stones and biliary disorders.

It is a pleasure to acknowledge the patient secretarial assistance of Barbara Tucker and Beryl Barbour, and the help and encouragement of Geoff Greenwood at Grune & Stratton, Ltd.

London 1984   **R. W. M.**

Contents

1
Introduction

Roger W. Motson

Why are gall-stones left behind in the common bile duct? The operative technique is standardized, per-operative cholangiography is widely used, and modern choledochoscopes allow us to inspect the interior of the common bile duct under direct vision. The incidence of retained stones has probably decreased over the last few decades but, even though surgeons are well aware of the problem, far too many stones are still overlooked. It is these stones that surgeons have failed to find that are euphemistically described as "retained" stones, with the implication that the fault lies with the common bile duct. It is a sad indictment of modern surgery that practitioners of the various techniques to remove retained stones have been able to accumulate huge numbers of cases in short periods of time. Burhenne reported a personal experience of 661 cases undergoing stone extraction via the T-tube tract in seven years,[1] and it took only four years for Safrany and colleagues to collect 3070 patients referred for endoscopic stone removal at 15 centres in Europe.[2]

Accurate estimates of the numbers of retained stones occurring annually are hard to obtain. In the United Kingdom approximately 40,000 cholecystectomies are performed each year.[3] Common bile duct stones will be present in approximately 12%, or 4800, of these cases who will in addition undergo a stone-positive common bile duct exploration (see Chapter 2, Table 2.1, p. 9). The total number of common bile duct explorations will of course be greater, depending on how readily individual surgeons explore the common duct. The negative exploration rate will be greatest when based on clinical criteria alone (history of jaundice, dilated common bile duct, wide cystic duct, small gall-bladder stones), and least when exploration is based on palpation of stones in the common duct and positive operative cholangiography. The incidence of retained stones varies greatly from surgeon to surgeon, ranging from a low of 1–2% to 10–15% or even higher. In the United States it is estimated that 12 million women and 4 million men have gall-stones. About 800,000 new cases of cholelithiasis occur each year.[4] Approximately 500,000 cholecystectomies are performed each year,[5] though even higher numbers, approaching 750,000 have also been suggested.[6] In Japan,[7] Scandinavia,[8] and South America[9] the prevalence of gallstones may be even higher than in either the United States or Great Britain.

Taking the lower United States estimate of 500,000 and the same 12% incidence of common duct stones, then 60,000 positive explorations will be performed each year. Again, there is great variation in the incidence of retained stones. The projected numbers for different average national incidences appear in Table 1.1. It is likely that the estimates for a 10% incidence are closest to what is actually occurring in practice across each country.

There is no question that in some cases exploration of the common bile duct is extremely difficult and taxes even the most experienced biliary surgeons. It is also clear that the greater numbers of stones that are present in the bile ducts, the greater the chances will be of leaving one or more stones behind.[10] However, retained stones are not confined to these difficult cases and far too many follow apparently straightforward common duct explorations at which relatively few stones are present. Some of these stones are not detected either because per-operative cholangiograms have not been performed or because the films that have been taken are of poor quality. Stones are present in the common bile duct with equal frequency whether the cholecystectomy is an elective operation or an emergency or urgent procedure for acute cholecystitis.[11] It is therefore important not to omit cholangiography in these cases unless common duct stones are palpable. In other cases there has been a failure to use available aids such as post-exploratory cholangiography or choledochoscopy to confirm complete clearance of the common duct before completing the operation. Retained stones detected on a cholangiogram one week post-operatively are detected seven days too late. Furthermore, in some patients with multiple stones insufficient consideration may have been given to the question of whether or not a duct drainage procedure, either choledochoduodenostomy or sphincteroplasty, is necessary. In addition, more recently, there has perhaps been some complacency during common duct exploration engendered by the knowledge that there

Table 1.1

Incidence of retained common duct stones.

Cholecystectomies per annum	Positive Common duct explorations	Retained stones per annum			
		5%	10%	15%	20%
U.K. 40,000	4,800	240	480	720	960
U.S.A. 500,000	60,000	3,000	6,000	9,000	12,000

are now a variety of techniques available to treat retained stones. It must be remembered, however, that none of these techniques can remove every stone. Most have a failure rate of 5–10% and each method has its own complications. The initial operation provides the surgeon with his best opportunity to clear the common duct of stones.

Most surgeons feel that their own personal incidence of retained stones is of an acceptably low level and is not a problem for them. This is because it may be one, two or more years between cases and, unless an accurate personal record is kept, individuals tend to forget exactly when a retained stone occurred or even that it occurred at all. The true incidence of common duct stones is in the order of 10–15% of all patients undergoing cholecystectomy and the mean value is 12%.[4] Figure 1.1 relates the frequency of cholecystectomy with the frequency of retained common duct stones and enables the reader to instantly estimate his own percentage incidence of retained stones. Most would agree that an incidence of 1 or 2% is excellent, 5% is good, 10% is average, and 20% or more is unacceptably high. If a retained stone occurs each year your incidence is too high unless you are performing 150–200 cholecystectomies annually — a very busy biliary practice. A surgeon who performs only 20 cholecystectomies a year would have to have no more than one retained stone in nine years to achieve better than a 5% incidence, and no more than one in 20 years to have an incidence as low as 2%. The majority of general surgeons are probably not performing cholecystectomy more often than once each week (U.K. 40,000 cholecystectomy per year by 1000 Consultant General Surgeons = 40 cholecystectomies per surgeon per year). Almost five years must elapse between one retained stone and the next to achieve a 5% incidence of retained stones. It can be seen how easy it is to underestimate one's incidence and an interval of several years between cases does not necessarily indicate good performance.

The efficacy of the various non-operative techniques for retained stones has greatly reduced the frequency with which surgery is required, but it should not be excluded from the treatment options. In reports on one non-operative technique or another comparison is often made to old surgical series with complications and failure rates which do not compare well with these new techniques. In an important paper, Girard and Le Gros reported the results of a series of re-operations for retained common duct stones between 1969 and 1979.[12] The ducts were cleared in 66 out of 69 patients, a success rate of 96% comparable with the various non-operative techniques. The three patients whose ducts were not cleared of stones each underwent a further exploration which was successful. There was no mortality, no major complications, and only minor complications in six (8·3%). Their series included 33 re-operations in patients aged over 60 years; mean post-operative stay was 10 days. It is against these surgical results that the non-

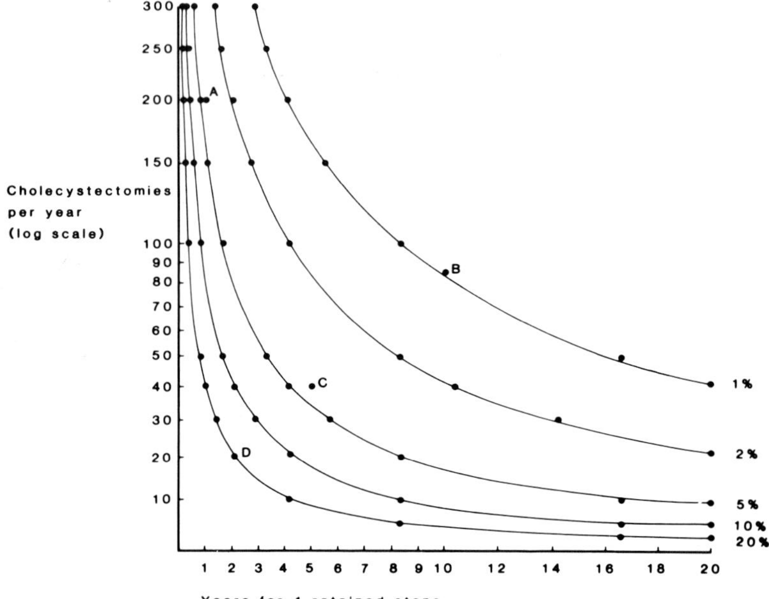

Fig. 1.1 To calculate incidence of retained stones. By relating the average number of cholecystectomies performed each year (y axis) to the number of years in which one retained stone occurs (x axis), it is possible to calculate the percentage incidence of retained stones. The curves shown have been calculated for a 12% incidence of common duct stones also present at the time of cholecystectomy.

Examples: (A) A busy unit with a particular interest in biliary surgery performs 200 cholecystectomies per year and has one retained stone per year; incidence $<5\%$. (B) A surgeon with an interest in biliary surgery performs 90 cholecystectomies per year and has one retained stone in 10 years; incidence 1%. (C) A general surgeon performs 40 cholecystectomies per year and has one retained stone in 5 years; incidence $<5\%$. (D) A surgeon performs 20 cholecystectomies per year and has a retained stone every 2 years; incidence 20%.

operative techniques must be compared. Difficulties can occur with the extraction techniques, particularly when the stones are large. In the majority of patients one of the non-operative approaches will be preferred. However, when this likely to be difficult consideration should be given to an elective operation to deal with the stones, rather than a much riskier emergency operation to treat haemorrhage or to disimpact an irretrievable stone basket following a failed non-operative attempt.

Another rarely employed treatment option is to do nothing at all. Data on this line of management are hard to come by but undoubtedly patients can harbour stones in the common bile duct without symptoms for many years. It is an option that should always be considered when one is faced with a very old patient in poor general health, particularly if there are few or no symptoms. This approach is unlikely to result in mortality and probably less than half of these patients will become symptomatic. If and when this occurs, interventional treatment can be reconsidered.

It must be the aim of every surgeon involved in biliary surgery to abolish the retained stone from his practice. We are now at a point where this should be an achievable goal. There are three distinct phases in surgery for common duct stones: pre-exploratory detection of stones, exploration and removal of stones, and post-exploratory examination to exclude retained stones. Attention to detail in each of these phases is essential if every stone present is to be detected and removed. The next three chapters examine each of these aspects. Operative cholangiography (Chapter 2) continues to have an important role in detecting unsuspected common duct stones, and equally importantly in avoiding unnecessary exploration of the common duct in patients with clinical indications for exploration. With careful attention to every detail the procedure adds little to the operative time and has a high diagnostic yield. Both supraduodenal and transduodenal techniques for common duct exploration are discussed in Chapter 3, together with the indications and techniques for drainage of the common duct by sphincteroplasty or choledochoduodenostomy. The use of the choledochoscope (Chapter 4) to exclude retained stones will continue to increase. When a choledochoscope is unavailable post-exploratory cholangiography (Chapter 2) should be employed.

When presented with a patient with a retained stone the surgeon is now faced with a wide choice of treatments (Table 1.2). The chapters in the

Table 1.2

Available treatments.

Infusions/Dissolution	Simple irrigation via T-tube
	Solvent infusion via T-tube
	Percutaneous/transhepatic solvent infusion
	Nasobiliary solvent infusion
	Oral stone dissolution agents
Extraction	Radiologically guided extraction via T-tube
	Choledochoscopic extraction via T-tube
	Endoscopic sphincterotomy alone
	Endoscopic sphincterotomy and stone extraction
Operation	Choledochotomy
	Sphincterotomy
	Sphincteroplasty
	Choledochoduodenostomy
	Choledochojejunostomy
None	Expectant treatment

second half of the book discuss each of the active treatments. When a stone is discovered on a post-operative cholangiogram simple flushing (Chapter 5) is well worth trying in almost every patient. If this is unsuccessful, and the T-tube is of adequate size, stone extraction either by steerable catheter under radiological control (Chapter 6) or by post-operative choledochoscopy (Chapter 7) should be employed after an interval of 5–6 weeks. At present these techniques are highly successful with few complications. If the T-tube is small, solvent infusion (Chapter 5) is simple but unpredictable in effect with a successful outcome in one-half to two-thirds of patients. When there is no T-tube present the choice lies between endoscopic sphincterotomy (Chapter 8), an interventional infusion technique (Chapter 5), oral dissolution therapy (Chapter 5), surgery (Chapter 9) or doing nothing. In most of these patients endoscopic sphincterotomy will be the preferred technique, but in some cases each of the other techniques will have a useful role.

REFERENCES

1. Burhenne HJ. Percutaneous extraction of retained biliary tract stones: 661 patients. Amer J Roentgenol 134: 889–898, 1980.
2. Safrany L. Endoscopic treatment of biliary-tract diseases. An international study. Lancet ii: 983–985, 1978.
3. Hospital in-patient inquiry, 1980; main tables. Department of Health and Social Security; Office of Population, Censuses and Surveys. London, HMSO: in press.
4. Small DM. The etiology and pathogenesis of gallstones. Advances in Surgery, Vol 10 (WP Longmire Jr, Ed). Chicago, Year Book, pp. 63–85, 1976.
5. Nakayama F, Miyake H. Changing state of gallstone disease in Japan. Composition of the stones and treatment of the condition. Amer J Surg 120: 794–799, 1970.
6. Torvik A, Hoivik B. Gallstones in an autopsy series. Incidence, complications and correlations with carcinoma of the gallbladder. Acta Chir Scand 120: 168–174, 1960.
7. Marinovic I, Guerra C, Larach G. Incidencia de litiasis biliar en material de autopsias y analisis de composicion de los calculos. Rev Med Chile 100: 1320–1327, 1972.
8. Way LW. Retained common duct stones. Symposium on Surgery of the Biliary Tree. Surg Clin N Amer 53: 1139–1148, 1972.
9. Wood M. Eponyms in biliary tract surgery. Amer J Surg 138: 746–754, 1979.
10. Way LW, Admirand WH, Dunphy JE. Management of choledocholithiasis. Ann Surg 176: 347–359, 1972.
11. Pitluk HC, Beal JM. Choledocholithiasis associated with acute cholecystitis. Arch Surg 114: 887–888, 1979.
12. Girard RM, Legros G. Retained and recurrent bile duct stones. Surgical or nonsurgical removal? Ann Surg 193: 150–154, 1981.

2
Operative Cholangiography

Roger W. Motson

Operative cholangiography was first performed by Mirizzi in 1931[1] and has since become an established part of biliary surgical practice.[2,3] The main purpose of the technique is to demonstrate common bile duct calculi at the time of cholecystectomy. In addition, the entire biliary tree can be visualized and anatomical variations are accurately delineated. Cholangiography is also valuable in other biliary operations for benign and malignant strictures, hepatic resections, etc.

A number of patients undergoing elective cholecystectomy will be known to harbour stones in the common bile duct following pre-operative endoscopic retrograde, percutaneous transhepatic or intravenous cholangiography. Intravenous cholangiography is performed relatively infrequently because a few patients react to the iodinated contrast medium. A protein electrophoretic strip should be performed routinely before every intravenous cholangiogram to detect the few patients who have an M-band monoclonal gammopathy in whom the risk of fatal reaction is high. It does not detect patients who will have minor reactions to the contrast medium. The technique is most reliable as a positive indicator, i.e. if a stone is demonstrated one will usually be found at exploration, but a normal result should be treated with some caution, particularly if some time has elapsed between the investigation and operation, or if opacification is poor. Poor visualization of the ducts has been a problem in about 15% of cases but recent improvements in the contrast media available have resulted in improved resolution on tomography.

The majority of patients will come to operation with a firm diagnosis of gall-bladder stones but without definite evidence for the presence or absence of stones in the common bile duct. Retained stones can only be prevented if all stones present are detected, and once detected are all then removed. The stones may be single or multiple, and in most patients are situated in the extrahepatic bile ducts with only occasional intrahepatic stones. In Caucasians the number of stones does not often exceed 10 and only rarely exceeds

20, but in the Orient, where recurrent pyogenic cholangitis is common, patients may present with the biliary tree packed with stones. Most common duct stones originate from the gall bladder and, therefore, are often facetted. Furthermore, in most cases on biochemical analysis the composition of the common bile duct stones is identical to gall-bladder stones from the same patient.[4] The incidence of common bile duct stones is difficult to ascertain accurately. In the series reported it is possible that some stones may have been missed, thus underestimating the true incidence; and many series include cases undergoing common bile duct exploration only, after cholecystectomy some years previously, and may therefore overestimate the true incidence. However, there is fairly close agreement between published series, with most giving an incidence of 10–15% (Table 2.1).

Some surgeons still remain sceptical as to the value of per-operative cholangiography,[11,12,15,18] and rely on duct palpation, a large diameter (> 12 mm) common bile duct, multiple small stones in the gall bladder, and a history of jaundice as indications for common duct exploration. There is considerable evidence that per-operative cholangiography reduces the negative duct exploration rate by demonstrating the absence of stones in patients fulfilling the above criteria for exploration.[8,24,25,26] In addition, per-operative cholangiography detects totally unsuspected stones in about 5% of patients without a history or operative indications for exploration (Table 2.2). False negative cholangiograms are very infrequent and are of the order of 0.7% with little variation between one author and another.[12,13,15,17,23,27,31–33] The incidence of falsely positive cholangiograms is much more variable and can often be related to technical shortcomings in the performance of the cholangiogram.[34] Gains (i.e. no exploration in patients with indications for exploration (15%) and unsuspected stones recovered (5%)) must be offset against losses (unnecessary explorations resulting from false positive cholangiograms). Good technique is essential in maintaining a positive balance. Opponents argue that the technique is tedious and time-consuming, that film quality is often poor, and that retained stones still occur. The criticisms of delay to the operation are particularly frequent when cholangiography is not "routine". The procedure can undoubtedly be performed quickly and efficiently if all concerned are familiar and practised at their respective roles. It is certainly true that retained stones still occur. Pre-exploratory per-operative cholangiography can only help to *prevent* retained stones in those few patients where stones are unsuspected and the common duct would otherwise not have been explored. In the remainder it is the quality of the common duct exploration and subsequent post-exploratory examination, not the pre-exploratory cholangiogram, that will determine if a stone is left behind. Pre-exploratory cholangiography can only be expected to indicate the presence or absence of

Table 2.1

Incidence of common duct stones (CDS) and common duct exploration (CDE) at cholecystectomy (CX).

Authors	Year	CX	CDE	CDE%	CDS	CDS/CDE%	CDS/CX%
Meyer et al.[5]	1967	1193	310	26.0	136	43.9	11.6
Schulenberg[6]	1969	1000	286	28.6	100	35.0	10.0
Wheeler et al.[7]	1970	201	47	23.5	34	72.3	16.9
Kakos et al.[8]	1972	753	188	25.0	116	61.7	15.4
Way et al.[9]	1972	952	200	21.0	130	65.0	13.7
Zimmerman-Nielsen et al.[10]	1975	1093	241	22.1	182	75.5	16.7
Mullen et al.[11]	1976	1000	110	11.0	57	51.8	10.1
Farha et al.[12]	1976	500	105	21.0	55	52.4	11.0
Faris et al.[13]	1976	400	109	27.3	78	71.6	19.1
Sugrue et al.[14]	1977	200	27	13.5	22	81.5	11.0
Stark and Loughry[15]	1980	440	47	10.6	30	63.8	6.8
Cranley and Logan[16]	1980	500	80	16.0	50	62.5	10.0
Pagana and Stahlgren[17]	1980	294	58	19.7	37	63.8	12.6
Cassie and Kapadia[18]	1981	382	25	6.5	23	92.0	6.0
Lygidakis[19]	1981	3710	430	11.6	347	80.7	9.4
Reasbeck[20]	1981	487	82	16.8	62	75.6	12.7
Rolfsmeyer et al.[21]	1982	340	54	15.9	38	70.4	11.2
Heuman et al.[22]	1982	1204	199	16.5	139	70.0	11.5
Levine et al.[23]	1983	585	97	16.6	139	70.0	11.5
TOTAL		15234	2695	17.7	1775	65.9	11.7

Table 2.2

Unsuspected common duct stones (CDS) demonstrated by per-operative cholangiography.

Authors	Year	No indication for choledochotomy	Unsuspected CDS No.	Unsuspected CDS %
Isaacs and Davies[28]	1960	87	7	8.0
Nienhuis[29]	1961	171	7	4.1
Letton and Wilson[30]	1966	105	6	5.7
Jolly et al.[31]	1968	380	24	6.3
Saltzstein et al.[26]	1973	427	8	1.8
Thurston[27]	1974	39	3	7.7
Farha et al.[12]	1976	395	26	6.6
Faris et al.[13]	1976	338	16	4.7
Wayne et al.[32]	1976	354	13	3.7
Stark and Loughry[15]	1980	322	3	0.9
Cranley and Logan[16]	1980	380	11	2.9
Pagana and Stahlgren[17]	1980	266	8	3.0
Levine et al.[23]	1983	130	4	3.1
TOTAL		3514	136	3.9

stones. It is a poor indicator of the number of stones, particularly when more than three of four stones are present.

Many factors contribute to successful operative cholangiography and several of these are outside the surgeon's control once the operation has started. Time spent on establishing efficient procedures with the radiological and theatre staff will be rewarded. Optimally performed cholangiography will produce satisfactory radiographs in 90% of cases.[24]

EQUIPMENT

Few surgeons will be fortunate enough to work in a purpose-built biliary surgery theatre, with image-intensifying x-ray equipment built into the operating table, providing facilities for screening and multiple spot films equal to an x-ray department, as described by Berci et al.[35] Most will be using general-purpose operating theatres and portable x-ray equipment. The theatre staff should ensure that there is free access for the mobile x-ray unit, with unobstructed doorways and floor space within the theatre. Ideally, the mobile x-ray unit should be in the theatre before the operation starts.

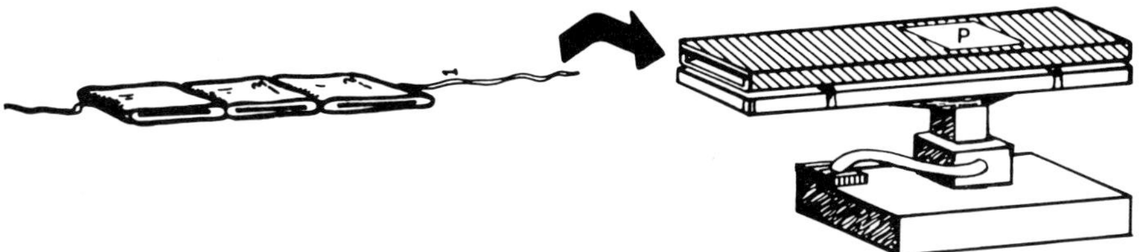

Fig. 2.1 Cassette tunnel for operative cholangiography. The shallow tunnel with a lead-screened top is placed on a standard operating table. Three cassettes are in place before the operation starts, with the first cassette under the radiolucent aperture (P). After each exposure successive cassettes are drawn into position. Markers (1, 2, 3) indicate when each cassette is aligned correctly. Further cassettes can be loaded without disturbing the sterile drapes and operating team.

A variety of systems exist to deliver the x-ray cassette under the patient, ranging from automated tables with a cassette carriage under the patient, to simple spacers which lift the mattress off the table base. Any system which requires access to the side of table, either to insert cassettes or to determine how far an automated cassette carriage should travel, disturbs the sterile drapes and operating team unnecessarily. A satisfactory and simple system is the end-loading tunnel first described by Samuel.[36] The patient is positioned accurately on top of a shallow wooden tunnel which has a 2 mm lead-screened top with a radiolucent aperture in the gall bladder area (Fig. 2.1). The x-ray cassettes are loaded into a linen runner which is inserted into the tunnel *before* the operation starts. Markers indicate when each film is under the radiolucent aperture and successive films can be drawn rapidly into place after each exposure. The films are withdrawn from the end of the table for processing. Further films for post-exploratory cholangiography can be loaded from the foot of the table without disturbing either the surgeon or assistants. The radiolucent aperture may be filled with a simple perspex sheet, the image intensifying grid or by an exposure-sensing plate which can be connected to the portable x-ray machine to give automated exposure control.

The terminal segment of the common bile duct overlies the vertebral column in some patients and this can cause stones to be missed. It should be routine procedure to tilt the patient to the right during cholangiography to avoid superimposition. It is customary for the intensifying grid to be orientated longitudinally in the cassette, parallel with the long axis of the table. Tilting will cause the grid apertures to be narrowed and picture quality may be lost. This potential problem is easily circumvented by arranging for the grid to be orientated transversely. Tilting may then occur without any effect on grid aperture (Fig. 2.2). Use of a single grid in the aperture of the

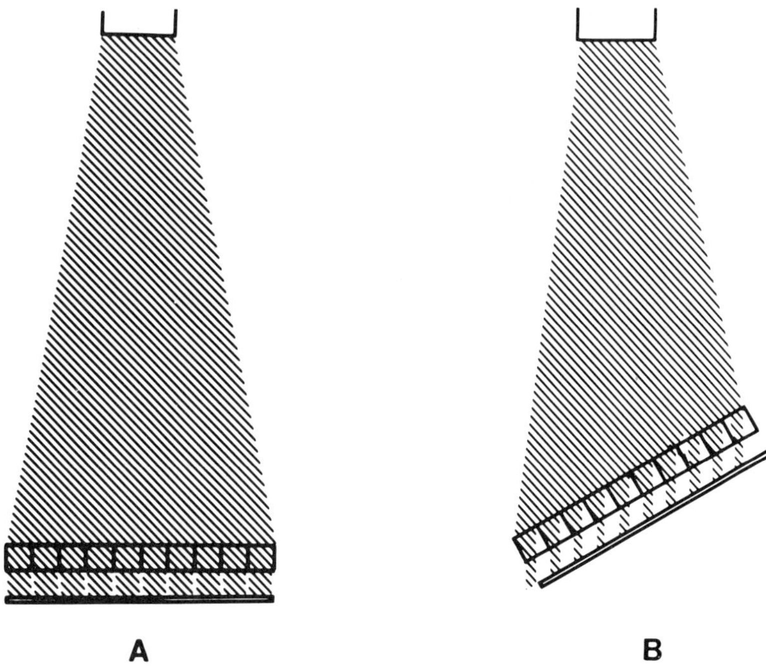

A   B

Fig. 2.2 Orientation of the image-intensifying grid. When the table is level the intensifying grid orientated longitudinally causes minimal interference with the x-ray beam. (A) When the table is tilted to separate the biliary tree from the lumbar spine considerable cut-off can occur. (B) This does not occur if the grid is orientated tranversely.

cassette tunnel avoids exposure variations which can occur when three different grids are used in the cassettes, and furthermore is economical with each grid costing £200.

It is particularly important that a senior radiographer is available for theatre work. It is unfair to the patient, the surgeon, and the radiographer if a junior unfamiliar with the equipment and theatre routine is assigned to these cases. Poor quality films may lead to unnecessary duct exploration or conceal a stone that is present. This makes it doubly important that cholangiograms are right first time, with the increased morbidity and mortality associated with common bile duct exploration. The gall bladder may have been removed by the time the films have been processed and there are often insidious pressures, which should be resisted, to accept less than perfect films. Film processing should take place within the theatre suite to avoid delay, and the chemicals must be checked regularly with test films if the dark room is not used frequently.

CYSTIC DUCT CHOLANGIOGRAPHY

It is axiomatic that the junction of the cystic duct with the common bile duct is clearly identified. Traction on gall-bladder forceps applied to Hartmann's pouch straightens and steadies the cystic duct. It is not necessary, in most cases, to ligate and divide the cystic artery within the triangle of Calot before proceeding to cholangiography. The proximal end of the cystic duct is closed most easily by a large tantalum clip (Ethicon Ligaclip or Weck Hemoclip) to prevent any further calculi leaving the gall bladder. Alternatively a ligature may be used though its placement and tying and clipping is a more time-consuming technique. A small incision is made in the cystic duct which is then probed to break down the spiral valve of Heister.

A wide variety of catheters are available made of metal,[37,38] polythene[39] and nylon.[40] The widely used Stoke-on-Trent cannula[40] tends to kink if it meets any resistance, and its plain unfinished tip is very prone to catching on the spiral valve. Olive-tipped ureteric catheters are easy to insert, and have centimetre calibration, but their opaque wall may conceal air bubbles; metal cannulae have the same disadvantage. The ideal catheter should be transparent, sufficiently rigid not to kink as it is inserted, with a smooth tip to aid insertion, and a collar to prevent accidental displacement. A catheter with these ideal specifications is now being produced by Portex Ltd. (Fig. 2.3).

The catheter is filled with saline to exclude all air bubbles and then inserted into the cystic duct. It may be held in position by thread[3] or rubber[41] ligature, tantalum clip[42,43] or a cholangiogram clamp.[44-46] Alternative techniques include the use of a modified Javid shunt[47] and a lymphangiogram cannula.[48] The cholangiogram clamp is a very lightweight artery forcep which has a right-angled tip with 6 and 7 French Gauge holes drilled in the jaws to hold the catheter in place without traumatizing the cystic duct (Figs. 2.4, 2.5). Usually the smaller hole closest to the tip of the instrument is used, but when a thick-walled duct is encountered the larger hole is used. The clamp may be applied with great accuracy since the surgeon's view is not obscured by his own hands as is so often the case when tying a ligature. Furthermore, the catheter is fixed with a single hand movement rather than the six to eight movements required to place and secure a ligature.

If the gall bladder and cystic duct cannot be identified easily, or the patient has undergone a cholecystectomy previously, then cholangiography can only be performed by direct puncture of the common bile duct. A butterfly 21 s.w.g. needle is frequently used, but there is a tendency for the needle to be displaced easily during injection of contrast and the dye extravasates. Modified Babcock[49] or fine artery forceps[50] hold the needle in place securely by grasping a small fragment of the duct wall thus securing the needle and preventing leakage.

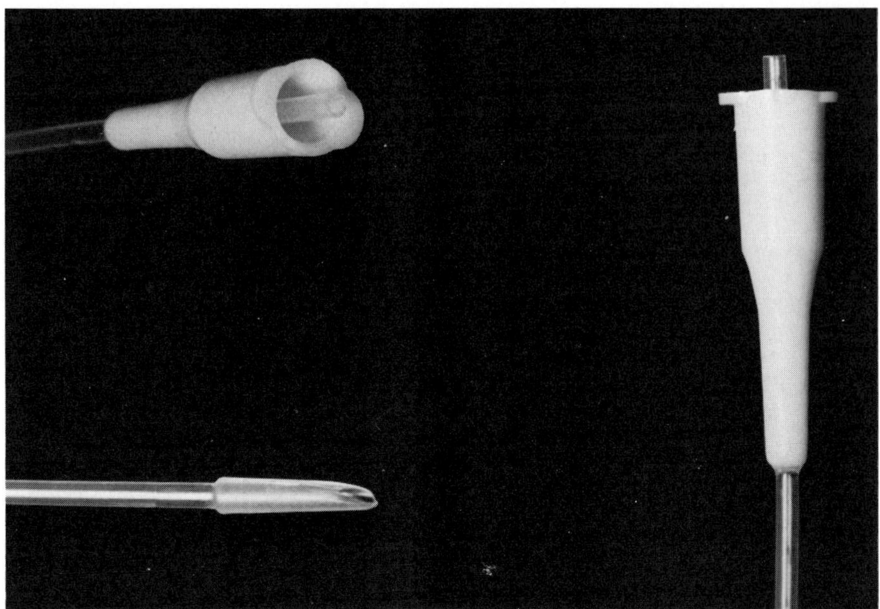

Fig. 2.3 Operative cholangiography catheter. The catheter is made of nylon which is extremely resistant to kinking, and has a bevelled beaded tip. The bevel makes insertion easy; once inserted the catheter is secured by a clamp or ligature and then drawn back into the cystic duct avoiding distortion of the common bile duct. The beaded tip prevents the catheter being accidentally withdrawn or dislodged. The nylon tube extends through the Luer–Lok hub, reducing the possibility of air entering the catheter as a syringe is connected. (Manufactured by Portex & Co., Hythe, Kent, U.K.)

A few millitres of saline are injected to confirm that the catheter is patent and that there is no leakage. The injection of saline also increases the pressure within the duct and aids retrograde flow of bile along the catheter when the saline-filled syringe is removed. A second syringe containing 25% Hypaque is then attached to the catheter. Great care should be taken to ensure that no air bubbles enter the system. The elasticity of the rubber bung within the syringe tends to draw air into the hub. When attaching the syringe to the catheter slight positive pressure should be applied so that a droplet of contrast bulges beyond the tip of the hub. More concentrated solutions of contrast should not be used because small stones can be concealed by a dense column of contrast in a large duct.[34] If the duct is particularly large the contrast medium should be diluted further with an equal volume of saline to produce a 12.5% solution.

When image intensification fluoroscopy is used small aliquots (1–2 ml) of

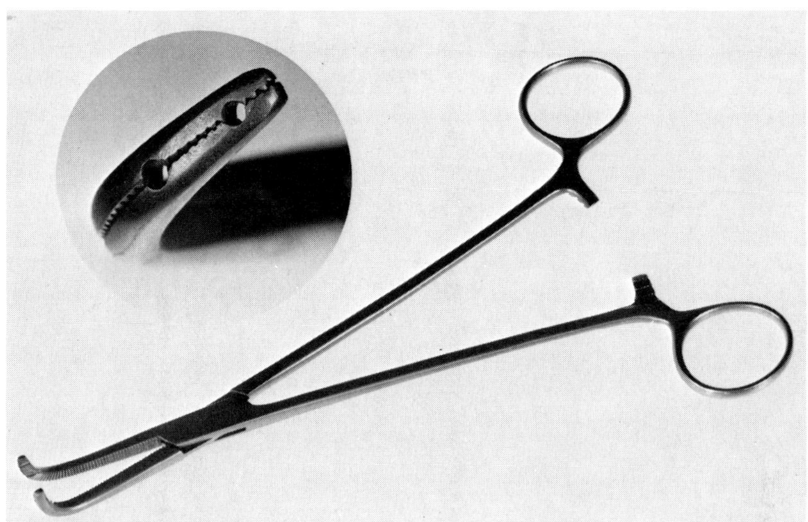

Fig. 2.4 Operative cholangiography clamp. The lightweight clamp holds the catheter securely in place occluding the cystic duct without damaging its wall. Normally the smaller (6 Fr.) hole closest to the tip of the instrument is used but when a thick-walled duct is encountered the larger (7 Fr.) hole is used. (Manufactured by Seward Surgical Ltd., London SE1 9UG, U.K., catalogue no. 630281.)

contrast are instilled, and the function of the sphincter of Oddi and emptying of the duct observed. One or two films should be taken to provide a permanent record. When fluoroscopy is not available three films should be taken. One–two millitres of contrast are instilled, and the first film taken during a brief period of apnoea. The initial injection must be limited to this small amount to prevent a flood of contrast into the duodenum obscuring the terminal segment of the common bile duct. Proximal filling can be encouraged in the second or third film by temporarily occluding bile duct by digital pressure below the catheter while the contrast medium is injected. Subsequent films are exposed after injection of a further 3–4 and 5–6 ml of contrast. The gall bladder is removed while the x-rays are processed. Exposure should only take place after, not during, the injection because the flow of contrast may set small stones in motion making them more difficult or impossible to see. Furthermore, exposure after injection allows the surgeon to move away from the patient, thereby minimizing his own exposure to x-rays.

Each cholangiogram series must be examined systematically for the following features:

1. filling of both left and right hepatic ducts;

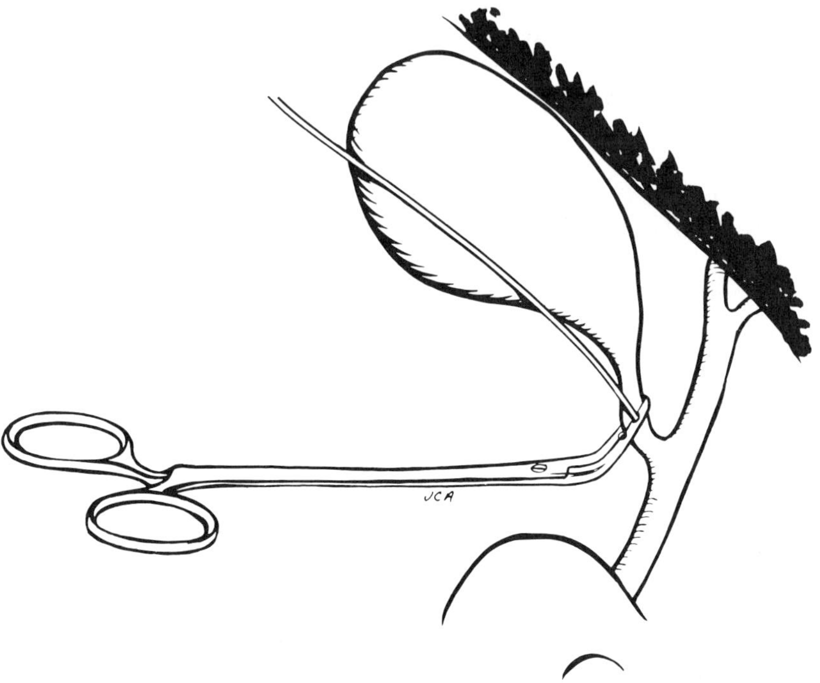

Fig. 2.5 Operative cholangiography clamp. After insertion of the cholangiogram catheter the cystic duct is cross-clamped under direct vision.

2. common bile duct diameter (normally < 12 mm);
3. presence or absence of filing defects;
4. a normal terminal segment;
5. free flow of contrast into the duodenum.

The cholangiogram may also demonstrate anatomical anomalies and abnormalities of cystic duct insertion. The cystic duct enters the common bile duct laterally at an exact right angle in only a proportion of cases. In others, the cystic duct may enter anteriorly, posteriorly or spiral around the common duct. It is difficult to ascertain the proportion of cases with each variant and there are considerable differences in the percentages of each in an anatomical series[51] compared with a radiological assessment.[52] It is more important to be aware of these variations and not to dissect the cystic duct to its termination. Such attempts in patients whose cystic duct has part of its course within the wall of the common bile duct may lead to the development of a subsequent stricture. Some errors are undoubtedly due to the surgeon not recognizing abnormalities that are present. Adherence to a strict routine when assessing films should minimize this sort of error, together with rejection of inadequate films. When doubts exist it can be helpful to obtain an immediate report by a radiologist.

POST-EXPLORATORY CHOLANGIOGRAPHY

At the conclusion of a common duct exploration the surgeon must ensure that the duct is actually free of stones. It has been shown clearly that omission of a post-exploratory examination will lead to a higher incidence of retained stones.[9] Choledochoscopy (Chapter 4) is the most convenient method, as it gives an "instant" answer before closing the common duct. If a choledochoscope is not available then a post-exploratory cholangiogram should be performed. A number of surgeons complain that the technique is valueless and confusing because of the presence of air bubbles, leakage from the choledochotomy, and spasm preventing free flow of contrast into the duodenum. Careful attention to technique can minimize these errors and give excellent results. Le Quesne and colleagues have achieved an incidence of retained stones of just one patient in a series of 109 common bile duct explorations in which 78 patients had stones recovered (incidence 1·3% of stone-positive explorations).[13]

Before common duct closure

Performing completion cholangiography before closure of the choledocho-tomy is attractive in that it avoids re-opening the incision when a stone is detected. A small Foley catheter is used. The tip of the catheter is trimmed off as the side hole may sometimes simulate a filling defect. One or two catheters are filled with saline and inserted into the choledochotomy. The balloons are inflated with a few millitres of saline to occlude the lumen of the common duct and prevent leakage from the choledochotomy[53,54] (Fig. 2.6). Twenty-five per cent Hypaque is then instilled and the cholangiograms taken. Recently a balloon T-tube has been devised to achieve the same purpose.[55] Contrast flows past the inflated balloon into both the proximal and distal biliary tree.

After common duct closure

Air within the long limb of the T-tube is a common cause of problems with completion cholangiography. Some surgeons rely on vigorous flushing with saline to clear the tube and bile duct of air bubbles though this is not always reliable. It will be found, almost invariably, by the time suturing of the choledochotomy has been completed that there will be a short column of bile

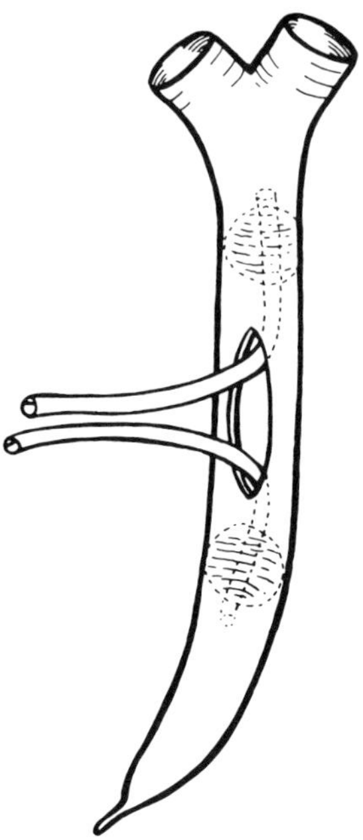

Fig. 2.6   Post-exploratory cholangiography before common duct closure. Two small Foley catheters with the tips trimmed off are inserted through the choledochotomy incision and gently inflated to maintain them in position. Contrast is then injected to fill the proximal and distal ducts.

in the T-tube close to the common duct (Fig. 2.7). Arterial forceps are used to cross-clamp the T-tube and column of bile below the meniscus, and a syringe of saline is then infused through a 23 s.w.g. needle into the T-tube just proximal to the forceps. All the contained air is flushed out as the long limb of the T-tube is completely filled with saline. A syringe of 25% Hypaque is then attached to the T-tube, the artery forceps removed, and the cholangiograms taken.[56] Larger volumes are needed as it takes approximately 10 ml of contrast to fill a 16 French gauge T-tube.

Interpretation of post-exploratory cholangiograms is really limited to the presence or absence of filling defects. It is quite common after passage of instruments through the ampulla that the cholangiogram shows no flow into the duodenum and the terminal segment is also not shown. These findings do not indicate an abnormal duct nor the presence of a stone as they do in a pre-exploratory film. The only reliable indication of a stone on a post-exploratory T-tube cholangiogram is the presence of a filling defect (Le Quesne, personal communication).

A large T-tube (16 or 18 Fr. gauge) should always be used to create a wide

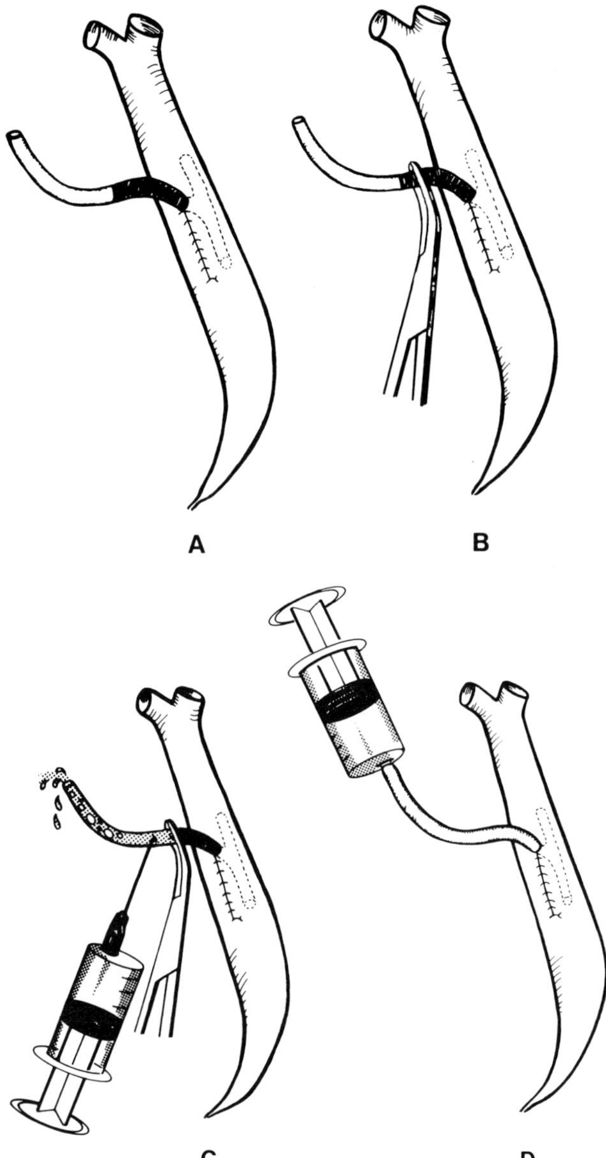

Fig. 2.7 Post-exploratory cholangiography after common duct closure. (A) By the time the choledochotomy incision has been closed some bile will have entered the T-tube. (B) The T-tube is cross-clamped across the column of bile. (C) A syringe of saline is then injected into the T-tube through a fine needle inserted just above the clamp, flushing air bubbles out of the end of the T-tube. (D) A syringe of contrast is then attached to the end of the T-tube and the clamp removed.

track which will allow insertion of stone-retrieval instruments, however unlikely a possibility this may seem. The back wall of the cross-bar can be trimmed away to produce a smaller intraductal segment. It is important that the T-tube is brought out without any intra-abdominal loops which would make subsequent instrumentation difficult.[57-59] Ideally, the T-tube should describe a smooth curve under the liver to emerge laterally. Use of a continuous suture (polyglycolic acid or polyglactin) produces a watertight closure, seems to have no disadvantage when compared with interrupted sutures, and greatly improves the quality of the post-exploratory cholangiogram.

Properly performed, pre-exploratory per-operative cholangiography remains a simple and effective method for detecting the presence or absence of common duct stones. It will lead to the recovery of unsuspected stones in about 5% of patients, and avoid unnecessary choledochotomy in about 15% of patients with clinical indications for exploration but normal cholangiograms. Common bile duct exploration is incomplete without a post-exploratory examination. Although choledochoscopy is increasingly taking over this role, a T-tube cholangiogram should be performed if a choledochoscope is not available. When no post-exploratory examination is performed the incidence of retained stones will be higher.

REFERENCES

1. Mirizzi PL. Operative cholangiography. Surg Gynecol Obstet 65: 702–710, 1937.
2. Hicken NF, Best RR, Hunt HB. Cholangiography. Visualization of the gallbladder and bile ducts during and after operation. Ann Surg 103: 210–229, 1936.
3. Le Quesne LP. Discussion of cholangiography. Proc R Soc Med 53: 852–855, 1960.
4. Bernhoft RA, Pelligrini CA, Motson RW et al. Composition and clinical features of common duct stones. Amer J Surg 148: 77–85, 1984.
5. Meyer KA, Capos NJ, Mittelpunkt AI. Personal experiences with 1261 cases of acute and chronic cholecystitis and cholelithiasis. Surgery 61: 661–668, 1967.
6. Schulenberg CAR. Operative cholangiography: 1,000 cases. Surgery 65: 723–739, 1969.
7. Wheeler MH, Raksasook S, Alexander Williams J. Operative cholangiography. Its effect on the practice of cholecystectomy. Brit Med J 4: 161–164, 1970.
8. Kakos GS, Tompkins RK, Turnipseed W et al. Operative cholangiography during routine cholecystectomy. A review of 3,012 cases. Arch Surg 104: 484–488, 1972.
9. Way LW, Admirand WH, Dunphy JE. Management of choledocholithiasis. Ann Surg 176: 347–359, 1972.
10. Zimmermann-Nielsen C, Dyreborg U, Madsen CM. Evaluation of peroperative cholangiography during cholecystectomy. Acta Chir Scand 141: 526–531, 1975.
11. Mullen JT, Carr RE, Rupnik EJ et al. 1,000 cholecystectomies, extraductal palpation, and operative cholangiography. Amer J Surg 131: 672–675, 1976.
12. Farha GJ, Pearson RN. Transcystic duct operative cholangiography. Personal experience with 500 consecutive cases. Amer J Surg 131: 228–231, 1976.

13. Faris I, Thomson JPS, Grundy DJ et al. Operative cholangiography: a reappraisal based on a review of 400 cholangiograms. Brit J Surg 62: 966–972, 1975.
14. Sugrue WJ, Stewart RJ, Pascoe DL et al. Operative cholangiography in two hundred consecutive cholecystectomies. NZ Med J 86: 470–471, 1977.
15. Stark ME, Loughry CW. Routine operative cholangiography with cholecystectomy. Surg Gynecol Obstet 151: 657–658, 1980.
16. Cranley B, Logan H. Exploration of the common bile duct — the relevance of the clinical picture and the importance of peroperative cholangiography. Brit J Surg 67: 869–872, 1980.
17. Pagana TJ, Stahlgren LH. Indications and accuracy of operative cholangiography. Arch Surg 115: 1214–1215, 1980.
18. Cassie GF, Kapadia CR. Operative cholangiography or extraductal palpation: an analysis of 418 cholecystectomies. Brit J Surg 68: 516–517, 1981.
19. Lygidakis NJ. Choledochoduodenostomy in calculous biliary tract disease. Brit J Surg 68: 762–765, 1981.
20. Reasbeck PG. The results of cholecystectomy at a district general hospital. A reappraisal of operative cholangiography. Ann R Coll Surg Eng 63: 359–362, 1981.
21. Rolfsmeyer S, Bubrick MP, Kollitz PR et al. The value of operative cholangiography. Surg Gynecol Obstet 154: 369–371, 1982.
22. Heuman R, Smeds S, Hellgren E et al. Evaluation of factors affecting the incidence of retained calculi in the bile ducts. Acta Chir Scand 148: 185–187, 1982.
23. Levine SB, Lerner HJ, Leifer ED et al. Intraoperative cholangiography. A review of indications and analysis of age–sex groups. Ann Surg 198: 692–697, 1983.
24. Holliday HJ, Farringer JL Jr, Terry RB et al. Operative cholangiography. Review of 7,529 operations on the biliary tree in a community hospital. Amer J Surg 139: 379–382, 1980.
25. Chapman M, Curry RC, Le Quesne LP. Operative cholangiography. An assessment of its reliability in the diagnosis of a normal , stone-free common bile duct. Brit J Surg 51: 600–601, 1964.
26. Saltzstein EC, Evani SV, Mann RW. Routine operative cholangiography. Analysis of 506 consecutive cholecystectomies. Arch Surg 107: 289–291, 1973.
27. Thurston OG. Nonroutine operative cholangiography. Arch Surg 108: 512–515, 1974.
28. Isaacs JP, Davies ML. Technique and evaluation of operative cholangiography. Surg Gynecol Obstet 111: 103–112, 1960.
29. Nienhuis LI. Routine operative cholangiography. An evaluation. Ann Surg 154: 192–202, 1961.
30. Letton AH, Wilson JP. Routine cholangiography during biliary tract operations: technic and utility in 200 consecutive cases. Ann Surg 163: 937–942, 1966.
31. Jolly PC, Baker JW, Schmidt HM et al. Operative cholangiography: a case for its routine use. Ann Surg 163: 551–565, 1968.
32. Wayne R, Cegielski M, Bleicher J et al. Operative cholangiography in uncomplicated biliary tract surgery. Review of 354 cholangiography studies in patients without indication of common duct pathology. Amer J Surg 131: 324–327, 1976.
33. Skillings JC, Williams JS, Hinshaw JR. Cost-effectiveness of operative cholangiography. Amer J Surg 137: 26–31, 1979.
34. Hall RC, Sakiyalak P, Kim SK et al. Failure of operative cholangiography to prevent retained common duct stones. Amer J Surg 125: 51–63, 1973.

35. Berci G, Steckel R. Modern radiology in the operating room. Arch Surg 107: 577–586, 1973.
36. Samuel E. Operative cholangiography. Brit J Radiol 32: 669–672, 1959.
37. Rabinov K, MacArthur J. Improved cannula instrument for operative cholangiography. Arch Surg 115: 229, 1980.
38. Berci G, Shore JM. Improved cannula for operative (cystic duct) cholangiography. Amer J Surg 137: 826–828, 1979.
39. Broome A, Jensen R, Thorne J. A new cholangiography catheter. Acta Chir Scand 142: 421–422, 1976.
40. Buchanan JMcK, Allen DS. Disposable cholangiogram cannula. Brit Med J 2: 448, 1969.
41. Goodman JM. Rubber ligature for cholangiographic catheter fixation. Amer J Surg 114: 972, 1967.
42. Shore JM, Berci G. A simple rapid technic for cystic duct cholangiography. Amer J Surg 123: 741–742, 1972.
43. Gunn A. The use of tantalum clips during operative cholangiography. Brit J Surg 67: 146, 1980.
44. Borge J. Operative cholangiography. New cholangiogram catheter clamp and improved technique. Arch Surg 112: 340–342, 1977.
45. Taufic M. A safe and secure technique of cystic duct catheterization. Arch Surg 114: 749–751, 1979.
46. Kidman DJ, Motson RW. Easier operative cholangiography. Aust NZ J Surg 49: 263–266, 1979.
47. Swenson WM. Cholangiography using a modified Javid shunt. Surg Gynecol Obstet 144: 925–926, 1977.
48. Devlin HB, Sahay AK, Tiwari PN et al. Cholecystectomy and a simple technique of operative cholangiography. Brit J Surg 65: 848–851, 1978.
49. Abbott AC. A new instrument for operative cholangiography. Surg Gynecol Obstet 119: 854–856, 1964.
50. Berci G, Hamlin JA. Re-exploration. The choledochocholangiogram. Operative Biliary Radiology (G Berci and JA Hamlin Eds). Baltimore, Williams & Wilkins, pp. 159–163, 1981.
51. Moosman DA, Carter FA. Prevention of traumatic injury to the bile ducts. Amer J Surg 82: 132–143, 1951.
52. Hamlin JA. Biliary ductal anomalies. Operative Biliary Radiology (G. Berci and JA Hamlin Eds). Baltimore, Williams & Wilkins, pp. 109–135, 1981.
53. Gunn AA. Cholecystectomy, cholecystostomy and exploration of the common bile duct. Operative Surgery, 3rd edn (CH Robb and R Smith Eds). London, Butterworths, p. 343, 1983.
54. Gervin AS, Fischer RP. Simple technique for operative assessment of retained stones in the common bile duct. Surg Gynecol Obstet 155: 251–252, 1983.
55. Kelly TR, Fink JA. A new inflatable T-tube for completion cholangiography. Surg Gynecol Obstet 158: 374–375, 1983.
56. van Heerden JA. A technique for T-tube cholangiography. Arch Surg 111: 85, 1976.
57. Mason RR. Dealing with residual bile duct stones. Brit Med J 4: 1788, 1978.
58. Motson RW. Dealing with residual bile duct stones. Brit Med J 1: 199, 1979.
59. Burhenne J. Nonoperative retained biliary tract stone extraction. A new roentgenologic technique. Am J Roentgenol 117: 383–399, 1973.

3

Exploration of the Common Bile Duct

Roger W. Motson

Cholecystectomy for gall-stones was first performed by Langenbuch in 1882,[1] and it was not long before surgeons found that they needed to explore the common bile duct. The first exploration is generally attributed to Thornton, who described two successful cases in 1887, in which stones were crushed and removed via a dilated cystic duct, and two further cases in 1889, in which the stones were removed through a choledochotomy.[2,3] Abbe,[4] Marcy,[5] and Courvoisier[6] all performed choledochotomy within a few months of Thornton, but Courvoisier was certainly the first to operate for a retained common duct stone in a patient who had previously undergone cholecystectomy.[6] Common duct exploration has continued to tax biliary surgeons ever since.[7,8] Exploration must be gentle, careful, unhurried, and absolutely meticulous. Furthermore, an exploration for common duct stones must be considered to be incomplete unless a post-exploratory examination either by choledochoscopy (Chapter 4) or cholangiography (Chapter 2) has been performed. Finally, one must consider whether or not there is a high risk of recurrent or retained stones, and hence if a duct drainage procedure is indicated. The common bile duct may be explored either via an incision in the supraduodenal portion of the duct or transduodenally.

TECHNIQUE

Supraduodenal exploration

The gall bladder usually will have been removed by the time per-operative cholangiograms are available to confirm, or indicate, the need for duct exploration. It is rarely possible to perform an adequate exploration through the cystic duct stump even if it is dilated. The cholangiogram catheter should therefore be removed and the cystic duct ligated. The right lateral aspect of the common duct will have been displayed during the identification of the cystic duct. Northover and Terblanche have shown very elegantly that the principal blood supply to the common duct is on its lateral aspects, with relatively few vessels anteriorly and posteriorly.[9] A little more dissection is therefore necessary to expose the anterior surface of the duct where the incision should be made. After insertion of stay sutures a vertical incision 1–2 cm long should be made in the duct immediately above the duodenum. The reasons for this are twofold: it is the most appropriate position for choledochoscopy, and also for choledochoduodenostomy if this should subsequently prove to be necessary.

A number of stones can be milked out of the common bile duct without the use of instruments, which minimizes trauma to the mucosa. Sandblom and Halabi were able to recover more than 50% of stones in this way.[10] Instrumental exploration of the proximal ducts is usually done first. A nearly straight pair of Desjardins forceps are ideal, and can be passed easily into both the right and left hepatic ducts. If stones are shown in the hepatic ducts on the cholangiogram, but not recovered with the forceps, then balloon catheters should be employed[11] either blindly or under direct vision via a choledochoscope, if available. Sometimes irrigation of the proximal ducts with saline via a small bore catheter will flush out additional stones. When this part of the exploration is complete it is often helpful to occlude the proximal ducts temporarily with a bile duct plug made from a half dental roll attached to a strong suture (Fig. 3.1). This prevents any stones disturbed in the exploration of the distal common bile duct from entering the proximal hepatic ducts. Furthermore, when the plug is removed at the end of the exploration the gush of bile that follows will sometimes carry small stone fragments from the proximal ducts which would not otherwise have been recovered. The distal common bile duct is undoubtedly more difficult to explore. Right-angled Desjardins forceps should be used first. If there is any difficulty in manipulating the instrument in the terminal part of the duct then the duodenum should be fully mobilized and further instrumentation carried out with the head of the pancreas between fingers and thumb. This enables the surgeon not only to feel where the tip of the forceps is, but also to exert a little traction to straighten the distal duct as it passes through the pancreas. It is important that the Desjardins forceps are very light in weight and have a freely moving joint. Heavy, stiff or more acutely angled instruments are useless. Bakes dilators should no longer form part of the instrumentation for common duct exploration, and evidence is accumulating from the increased use of endoscopic cholangiography that a number of choledochoduodenal fistulae are caused by these instruments when used for common duct exploration.[12–14] The balloon probe is also useful in recovering stones from the distal duct. Finally a soft catheter is passed down the duct. An 8 Fr gauge nasopharyngeal suction catheter (Vygon 533) or infant feeding tube (Warne WSP 6134) is ideal for irrigation. If the tip of the catheter passes into the

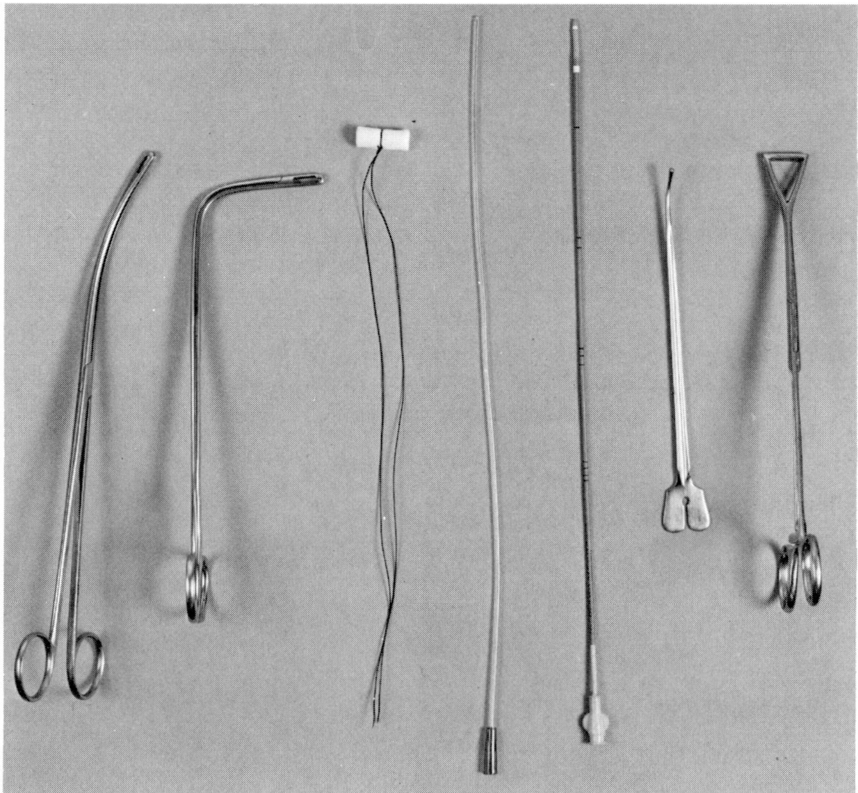

Fig. 3.1 Instruments for common bile duct exploration. Left to right: nearly straight Desjardins forceps, right-angled Desjardins forceps, half dental roll, soft polythene irrigation catheter, balloon catheter, grooved common bile duct sound, and Duval's forceps.

duodenum and is then flushed with saline, none of the irrigation fluid will escape from the choledochotomy. Irrigation is continued and the catheter is gently drawn back. As soon as the tip returns through the ampulla, fluid starts to escape from the choledochotomy. One can then irrigate vigorously, confident that the whole of the distal duct is being irrigated back towards the incision from the ampulla.

On completion of the exploration it is essential that the surgeon makes a post-exploratory examination either by cholangiography or choledochoscopy. Choledochoscopy, if available, is preferable because retained stones can be detected without any delay for the taking and processing of x-rays. If a choledochoscope is unavailable, cholangiography should be performed, since retained stones occur more frequently when there is no post-exploratory procedure.[15] The common bile duct is closed conventionally over a T-tube, though some surgeons prefer to close the duct primarily and rely on a drain near the duct which is removed after a few days. It is argued that this avoids T-tube-related complications, lowers the incidence of wound infection, and shortens hospital stay, without any increase in mortality.[16] It is, however, possible even with the most careful exploration to induce spasm of the sphincter of Oddi, which may result in leakage from the suture line, and a subhepatic collection of bile. Furthermore, this technique denies the easy post-operative access to the bile duct afforded by the T-tube tract for radiography and flushing, dissolution, or extraction of a retained stone should this subsequently prove to be necessary. On balance, the benefits of a T-tube probably outweigh its disadvantages for the majority of surgeons, apart from experienced choledochoscopists who can be very confident that the ducts are clear.

Transduodenal exploration

The peritoneum is incised on the lateral side of the duodenum, and the second part of the duodenum and the head of pancreas fully mobilized. It is well worthwhile spending a minute or two extra at this stage to ensure full mobilization which will make all the subsequent steps easier.

Accurately identifying the ampulla before opening the duodenum can be difficult, but when this can be achieved it means that only a short duodenotomy incision is necessary. If the ampulla is prominent it can be palpated. Alternatively, the cholangiogram catheter, a gum elastic bougie[17] or a Fogarty balloon catheter[18] can be introduced through the cystic duct and advanced through the ampulla to aid its identification, provided that there is no impacting stone. The duodenotomy is made in the long axis of the duodenum on its lateral border and the ampulla is then identified. If a catheter or bougie has not been advanced through the ampulla, infusion of saline through the cholangiogram catheter may aid identification and, once identified, Duval's forceps can be useful in maintaining exposure. A grooved director is passed through the ampulla into the common bile duct and an incision is then made at the upper border of the ampulla with a scalpel or Pott's angled scissors. Bile escapes immediately and the duct can then be explored with the nearly straight Desjardins forceps, balloon probes, and irrigation catheters. For sphincteroplasty, mucosal apposition is achieved using interrupted sutures between the duodenal wall and bile duct. A 000 Dexon or Vicryl suture is most suitable. Particular attention is paid to tying the apical suture (Fig. 3.2). Most surgeons exploring the duct in this manner do not use a T-tube drain, arguing that it is unnecessary and only increases

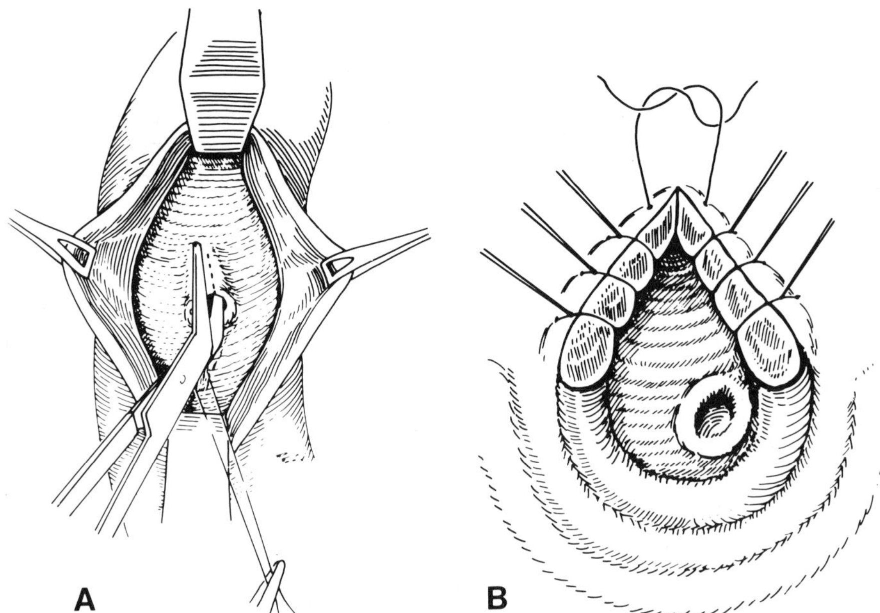

Fig. 3.2 Sphincteroplasty. (A) The sphincter of Oddi is divided with Pott's angled scissors. (B) Mucosal–mucosal apposition is achieved using interrupted sutures, with particular attention being paid to the apical suture. (Reproduced with permission from Dr R. E. Hermann and Annals of Surgery.)

complications. Furthermore, it is claimed that if a stone should have been overlooked it will escape through the open ampulla, and therefore the access to the duct provided by a T-tube is unnecessary. This is probably correct in the great majority of cases. In Austin Jones' series of 211 cases, when a T-tube was used only five stones were found on post-operative cholangiography.[19] All were flushed through easily into the duodenum.

There is much greater debate as to whether, after incising the sphincter, the cut edges should be left alone — sphincterotomy;[20] or whether mucosa-tomucosa suture is necessary — sphincteroplasty.[19,21] Strong views in favour of each have been advanced by their respective proponents, the former arguing that suture is not only unnecessary but risks damage to vessels or the pancreatic duct, and the latter arguing that without suturing, the incision closes down rapidly, and that extravasation of bile into the retroperitoneal tissues may sometimes occur. Surgeons who perform sphincterosplasty almost certainly make a more extensive incision in the knowledge that they are going to suture the duodenum and common duct together, whereas surgeons performing sphincterotomy must ensure that they do not breach the duodenal wall completely. The end result in sphincteroplasty is complete division of the spincter of Oddi, whereas in sphincterotomy some of the most proximal sphincter muscle fibres will be spared. It is this, rather than any failure of sphincterotomy to provide adequate division of the sphincter, that accounts for a common duct pressure increase in response to morphine, which is similar to, though lower than, normal after sphincterotomy, but which is only very transient after sphincteroplasty.[19] There has been much experience gained using sphincterotomy at The London Hospital, and there is no doubt that the technique provides good access to the common duct.[20,22] Post-operative endoscopic studies performed between four months and nine years later in 13 patients showed that the sphincterotomy remained widely open in nine, with continuous flow of bile in ten. In the remaining three patients, bile flowed intermittently similar to normals.[22] Endoscopic sphincterotomy, which resembles surgical sphincterotomy more closely than sphincteroplasty, has not yet been shown to have a high retain stenosis rate.

Overall, it seems that the differences between sphincterotomy and sphincteroplasty may be rather fewer than have previously been thought.

Combined exploration

When both supra- and transduodenal approaches are used together to explore the duct the morbidity in most series is higher.[20,23] This is not altogether surprising, as one would expect the complications of the two procedures together to be greater than either one alone. Furthermore, the fact that a combined approach was necessary usually indicates that difficulties have been encountered, and that the exploration may well have been traumatic, thereby making these patients a higher risk group. It is probably wise not to persist too long with an unsuccessful supraduodenal exploration. Aubrey and Edwards have reported very satisfactory results when employing combined exploration on this basis.[24]

On completion of any common duct exploration it is important to consider whether or not the patient would benefit from a duct drainage procedure. If there are very many stones, and hence a higher than normal likelihood of retained stones, if the operation is a re-exploration for a retained stone after previous cholecystectomy, if there is biliary sludge within the bile duct, if the patient is old or a particularly high operative risk for further surgery, then a duct drainage procedure may be appropriate.

If duct drainage is necessary, the choice lies between transduodenal sphincterotomy or sphincteroplasty as described above, or a side-to-side choledochoduodenostomy. Sphincterotomy and sphincteroplasty have the advantage of dependent drainage by gravity but are technically more difficult to perform, particularly for surgeons who do not carry out one or other of these procedures regularly, whereas choledochoduodenostomy[25,26] between an incised second part of duodenum and an already opened supraduodenal common duct is quick and easy to perform.

Choledochoduodenostomy

A vertical incision, at least 2–2.5 cm long, is made in the lowest part of the supraduodenal common bile duct. The duodenum is mobilized so that it can be "rolled up" over the common duct without tension. The direction of the duodenal incision is not critical. Some surgeons always make transverse and others always longitudinal incisions. It is probably best to see how the duodenum lies over the common duct and to make the incision in the direction that will lie in apposition to the choledochotomy with the least tension. A double-needled suture is ideal for choledochoduodenostomy (e.g. 00 Dexon, 7265.51). Starting within the duodenum, the suture passes into and out of the bile duct at the lower end of the choledochotomy and through the duodenal wall to be tied within the duodenal lumen. A continuous one-layer technique is employed and is completed by tying the two ends of the suture at the upper end of the choledochotomy (Fig. 3.3).

Choledochoduodenostomy has, in general, been more popular in Europe than in the United States. The operation was first performed by Riedel in 1888,[27] and popularized by Sasse in 1913.[28] The principal criticisms of the operation are its rather unphysiological route of drainage, and the accumulation of food debris in the distal common bile duct leading to pain and cholangitis — the so-called "sump" syndrome. Although this does occur sometimes the incidence is very low. If an adequate stoma is formed this complication should not occur, as food debris entering through a large stoma will easily escape again. It is only when the stoma is small or stenotic that symptoms are likely to occur. Experimental work in dogs, by Madden, has shown that cholangitis does not occur even when the common bile duct is anastomosed to the colon, provided that the stoma is large and stenosis does not occur.[26] Reflux of duodenal contents will also occur in patients who have undergone sphincteroplasty but again, symptoms do not occur unless there is stenosis.

In patients from the Orient, where the intrahepatic ducts may be packed with stones, residual stones may be almost inevitable. An ingenious modification of choledochojejunostomy has been devised by Peng and colleagues with a blind loop placed subcutaneously (Fig. 3.4). This allows access to the biliary tree without further laparotomy. The blind stoma can be opened under local anaesthetic and a choledochoscope inserted to retrieve stones from the hepatic ducts.[29]

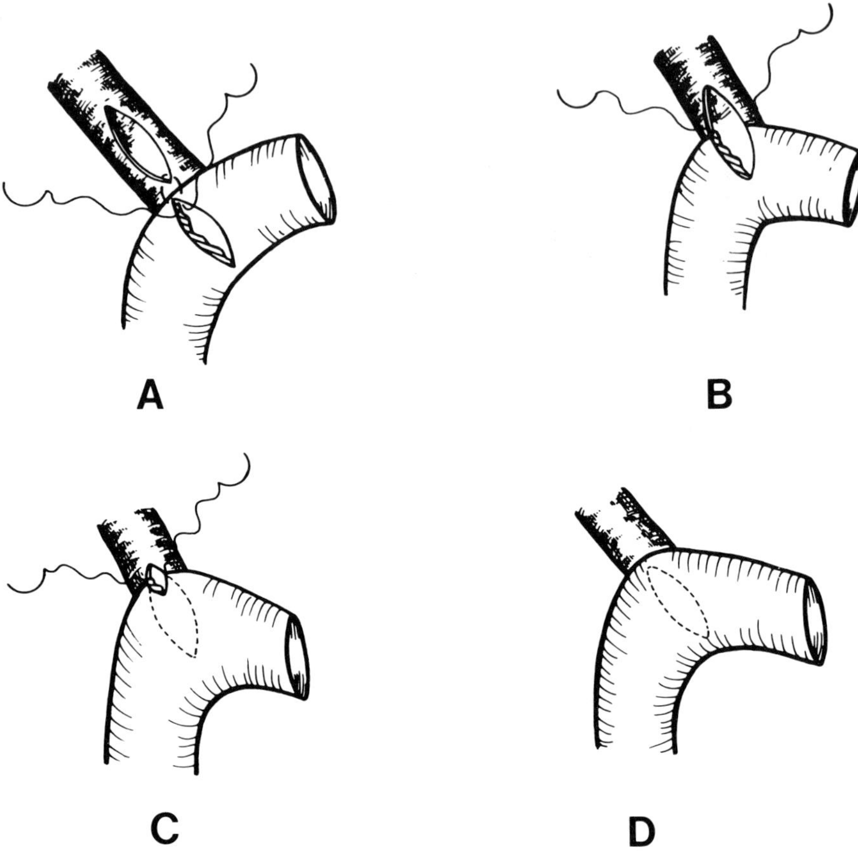

Fig. 3.3   Choledochoduodenostomy. Incisions 2.5 cm long are made in the supraduodenal common bile duct and duodenum. (A) A double-armed suture is used, starting within the duodenum, to make a continuous one-layer anastomosis. (B, C, D) As the anastomosis progresses, the duodenum "rolls up" over the duct.

Most published series contain a mixture of cases, mainly comprising patients in whom common duct exploration was performed at the same time as cholecystectomy, and a smaller number of cases undergoing a second or third exploration of the common duct alone. There is no doubt that the experienced surgeons who have a particular interest in one technique can achieve excellent results with low mortality and few complications (Tables 3.1–3.3), but the experience of others has not always matched up to this.[51]

Sphincterotomy and sphincteroplasty are particularly indicated for stones impacted at the lower end of the common bile duct, and for ampullary stenosis. They are much less satisfactory, and indeed are contra-indicated in

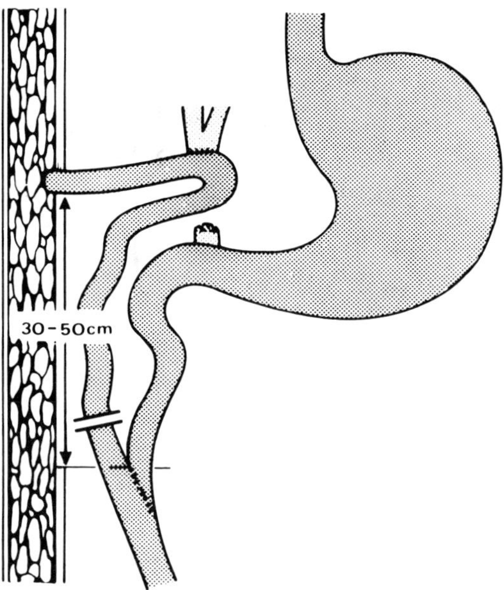

Fig. 3.4 Peng's operation for patients whose biliary tree is packed with stones. Hepaticojejunostomy is modified by a blind jejunal loop fixed subcutaneously. If further stones form, the loop may be entered under local anaesthesia and a flexible choledochoscope introduced to retrieve stones from the intrahepatic ducts. (Reproduced with permission from Dr S. Y. Peng and Annals of the Royal College of Surgeons of England.)

Table 3.1

Transduodenal sphincterotomy.

Authors	Year	No. cases	Mortality		Cholangitis	
			No.	%	No.	%
Thomas et al.[30]	1971	53	4	7.6	—	—
Stuart and Hoerr[17]	1972	18	1	5.6	—	—
Peel et al.[22]	1974	82	2	2.4	0	0.0
Partington[31]	1977	47	2	4.3	—	—
Vellacott and Powell[23]	1979	32	3	9.4	1	3.1
Panahy and Ritchie[32]	1982	109	2	1.8	1	0.9
Peel[33]	1984	83	0	0.0	3	3.6
TOTAL		424	14	3.3	5	1.6

Table 3.2

Transduodenal sphincteroplasty.

Authors	Year	No. cases	Mortality		Cholangitis	
			No.	%	No.	%
Stefanini et al.[34]	1974	712	7	1.1	—	—
Rutledge[35]	1976	60	0	0.0	—	—
Partington[31]	1977	87	2	2.3	—	—
Jones[19]	1978	312	3	1.0	—	—
Vogt and Hermann[36]	1981	37	0	0.0	—	—
Choi et al.[37]	1982	42	1	2.4	3	7.1
Strom and Stone[18]	1982	123	3	2.4	—	—
Leckie et al.[38]	1982	21	1	4.8	—	—
Nardi et al.[39]	1983	95	4	4.2	—	—
Carter[40]	1983	212	12	5.7	0	0.0
Antrum and Hall[41]	1984	118	3	2.5	—	—
TOTAL		1819	36	2.0	3	1.2

Table 3.3

Choledochoduodenostomy.

Authors	Year	No. cases	Mortality		Cholangitis	
			No.	%	No.	%
Madden et al.[26]	1970	100	4	4.0	0	0.0
Thomas et al.[30]	1971	57	2	3.5	—	—
Stuart and Hoerr[17]	1972	13	0	0.0	—	—
Degenshein[42]	1974	175	7	4.0	2	1.1
Rutledge[35]	1976	13	0	0.0	1	7.7
Keighley et al.[43]	1976	28	0	0.0	—	—
Schein and Gliedman[44]	1978	100	3	3.0	0	0.0
Kaminski et al.[45]	1979	25	1	4.0	—	—
Lygidakis[46]	1981	342	0	0.0	0	0.0
Vogt and Hermann[36]	1981	88	4	4.6	4	4.6
Lygidakis[47]	1982	92	0	0.0	—	—
de Almeida[4-8]	1984	70	1	1.4	—	—
TOTAL		1103	22	2.0	7	0.9

the presence of a peri-ampullary duodenal diverticulum or if there are very large common duct stones to be removed. These techniques also provide access to the pancreatic duct, which may be cannulated and operative pancreatography performed. Some surgeons attach particular importance to the septum between biliary and pancreatic ducts, and believe this should be divided in some cases.[46,47] This view is particularly espoused in the United States, where some patients undergo sphincteroplasty for pancreatitis or post-cholecystectomy pain, as well as for common duct stones.[48,49] Division of the septum is probably more appropriate in these cases than in patients who only have common duct stones.

Although there has now been much experience of sphincterotomy, only one prospective randomized trial of sphincteroplasty and choledochoduodenostomy has been performed.[50] In this study patients underwent either choledochotomy and T-tube drainage, sphincteroplasty, or choledochoduodenostomy. Approximately 40 patients were allocated to each group. Early morbidity and mortality, and late complications were lowest in the choledochoduodenostomy group.

The various approaches to the common bile duct, however, should not be regarded as competitors but as complementary to one another. In most patients, a supraduodenal choledochotomy with confirmatory choledochoscopy will be perfectly satisfactory. Stones impacted at the lower end of the duct are best approached transduodenally. If a duct drainage procedure is necessary there is little to choose between an adequate choledochoduodenostomy, transduodenal sphincterotomy or sphincteroplasty.

REFERENCES

1. Langenbuch C, Berl Klin Wehirschr 19: 725, 1882; cited by Maingot R. Abdominal Operations, Vol 1, 6th edn, New York, Appleton-Century-Crofts, p. 985, 1974.
2. Thornton JK. Two cases of cholecystostomy. Brit Med J 2: 1148–1150, 1887.
3. Thornton JK. Observations on additional cases illustrating hepatic surgery. Lancet i: 763, 1891.
4. Abbé R. Surgery of gallstone obstruction. Med Rec 43: 548–552, 1893.
5. Marcy HO. Surgical relief for biliary obstruction. J A M A 15: 887–894, 1890.
6. Courvoisier L. Casuistisch-Statistische Beitrage zur Pathologie und Chirurgie der Gallenwege. Leipzig: Vogel, pp. 280–281, 1890.
7. Editorial. Routine operative cholangiography. Lancet i: 1379– 1380, 1970.
8. Bevan PG. The elusive stone. Brit Med J 284: 1139–1140, 1982.
9. Northover JMA, Terblanche J. A new look at the arterial supply of the bile duct in man and its surgical implications. Brit J Surg 66: 379–384, 1979.
10. Sandblom P, Halabi M. Atraumatic removal of common duct stones. Surg Gynecol Obstet 139: 249–251, 1974.

11. Fogarty TJ, Krippaehne WW, Dennis DL et al. Evaluation of an improved operative technic in common duct surgery. Amer J Surg 116: 177–183, 1968.
12. Ikeda S, Okada Y. Classification of choledochoduodenal fistula diagnosed by duodenal fiberscopy and its etiological significance. Gastroenterology 69: 130–137, 1975.
13. Hunt DR, Blumgart LH. Iatrogenic choledochoduodenal fistula: an unsuspected cause of post-cholecystectomy symptoms. Brit J Surg 67: 10–13, 1980.
14. Martin DF, Tweedle DEF. The aetiology and significance of choledochoduodenal fistula. Brit J Surg 71: 632–634, 1984.
15. Way LW, Admirand WH, Dunphy JE. Management of choledocholithiasis. Ann Surg 176: 347–359, 1972.
16. Lygidakis NJ. Choledochotomy for biliary lithiasis: T-tube drainage or primary closure. Effects on postoperative bacteremia and T-tube bile infection. Amer J Surg 146: 254–256, 1983.
17. Stuart M, Hoerr SO. Late results of side to side choledochoduodenostomy and of transduodenal sphincterotomy for benign disorders. A twenty year comparative study. Amer J Surg 123: 67–72, 1972.
18. Strom PR, Stone HH. A technique for transduodenal sphincteroplasty. Surgery 92: 546–549, 1982.
19. Jones SA. The prevention and treatment of recurrent bile duct stones by transduodenal sphincteroplasty. World J Surg 2: 473–485, 1978.
20. Peel ALG, Bourke JB, Hermon-Taylor J et al. How should the common bile duct be explored? Ann R Col Surg Eng 56: 125–134, 1975.
21. Jones SA, Steedman RA, Keller TB et al. Transduodenal sphincteroplasty (not sphincterotomy) for biliary and pancreatic disease. Amer J Surg 118: 292–306, 1969.
22. Peel ALG, Hermon-Taylor J, Ritchie HD. Technique of transduodenal exploration of the common bile duct. Duodenoscopic appearances after biliary sphincterotomy. Ann R Coll Surg Eng 55: 236–244, 1974.
23. Vellacott KD, Powell PH. Exploration of the common bile duct: a comparative study. Brit J Surg 66: 389–391, 1979.
24. Aubrey DA, Edwards JL. The selective use of combined supraduodenal and transduodenal exploration of the common bile duct. Brit J Surg 65: 246–251, 1978.
25. Johnson AG, Rains AJH. Prevention and treatment of recurrent bile duct stones by choledochoduodenostomy. World J Surg 2: 487–496, 1978.
26. Madden JL, Chun JY, Kandalaft S et al. Choledochoduodenostomy. An unjustly maligned surgical procedure? Amer J Surg 119: 45–54, 1970.
27. Riedel BMCL. Erfahrungen uber die Gallensteinkrankheit mit und ohne Icterus. Berl Hischwald p. 116, 1892.
28. Sasse F. Über choledocho-duodenostomie. Arch Klin Chir 100: 969, 1913.
29. Peng SY, Yue MK, Qi VJ et al. Aspects of treatment at the Zhejiang Medical College, China. Ann R Coll Surg Eng 65: 50–51, 1983.
30. Thomas CG Jr, Nicholson CP, Owen J. Effectiveness of choledochoduodenostomy and transduodenal sphincterotomy in the treatment of benign obstruction of the common duct. Ann Surg 173: 845–856, 1971.
31. Partington PF. Twenty-three years of experience with sphincterotomy and sphincteroplasty for stenosis of the sphincter of Oddi. Surg Gynecol Obstet 145: 161–168, 1977.
32. Panahy C, Ritchie HD. Personal communication, 1983.
33. Peel ALG. Personal communication, 1984.

34. Stefanini P, Carboni M, Patrassi N et al. Transduodenal sphincteroplasty: its use in the treatment of lithiasis and benign obstruction of the common duct. Amer J Surg 128: 672–677, 1974.
35. Rutledge RH. Sphincteroplasty and choledochoduodenostomy for benign biliary obstructions. Ann Surg 183: 476–487, 1976.
36. Vogt DP, Hermann RE. Choledochoduodenostomy, choledochojejunostomy or sphincteroplasty for biliary and pancreatic disease. Ann Surg 193: 161–168, 1981.
37. Choi TK, Lee NW, Wong J et al. Extraperitoneal sphinteroplasty for residual stones, an update. Ann Surg 196: 26–29, 1982.
38. Leckie PA, Schmidt N, Taylor R. Impacted common bile duct stones. Amer J Surg 143: 540–541, 1982.
39. Nardi GL, Michelassi F, Zannini P. Transduodenal sphincteroplasty. 5–25 year follow-up of 89 patients. Ann Surg 198: 453–461, 1983.
40. Carter AE. The transduodenal per-ampullary approach to common bile duct calculi. Ann R Coll Surg Eng 65: 183–184, 1983.
41. Antrum RM, Hall R. Transduodenal sphincteroplasty: an analysis of 118 consecutive cases. Brit J Surg 71: 446–448, 1984.
42. Degenshein GA. Choledochoduodenostomy: an 18 year study of 175 consecutive cases. Surgery 76: 319–324, 1974.
43. Keighley MRB, Burdon DW, Baddeley RM et al. Complications of supraduodenal choledochotomy: a comparison of three methods of management. Brit J Surg 63: 754–758, 1976.
44. Schein CJ, Gliedman ML. Choledochoduodenostomy as an adjunct to choledocholithotomy. Surg Gynecol Obstet 146: 25–32, 1978.
45. Kaminski DL, Barner HB, Codd JE et al. Evaluation of the results of external choledochoduodenostomy for retained, recurrent, or primary common duct stones. Amer J Surg 137: 162–166, 1979.
46. Lygidakis NJ. Choledochoduodenostomy in calculous biliary tract disease. Brit J Surg 68: 762–765, 1981.
47. Lygidakis NJ. Surgical approaches to postcholecystectomy choledocholithiasis. Arch Surg 117: 481–484, 1982.
48. de Almeida AM, Cruz AG, Aldeia FJ. Side-to-side choledochoduodenostomy in the management of choledocholithiasis and associated disease. Amer J Surg 147: 253–259, 1984.
49. Cave-Bigley DJ, Aukland P, Kane JF et al. Transduodenal exploration of the common bile duct in a district general hospital. Ann R Coll Surg 66: 187–189, 1984.
50. Moody FG, Berenson MM, McCloskey D. Transampullary septectomy for post-cholecystectomy pain. Ann Surg 186: 415–423, 1977.
51. Moody FG, Becker JM, Potts JR. Transduodenal sphincteroplasty and transampullary septectomy for postcholecystectomy pain. Ann Surg 197: 627–636, 1983.
52. Lygidakis NJ. Prospective randomised study of recurrent choledocholithiasis. Surg Gynecol Obstet 155: 679–684, 1982.

4

Operative Choledochoscopy

Brian S. Ashby and Roger W. Motson

Choledochoscopy is the visual examination of the interior of the bile ducts during or after surgical exploration of the common and hepatic ducts, most commonly for gall-stones. Operative choledochoscopy, discussed in this chapter, may be either exploratory, when the choledochoscope is used as the exploring surgical instrument replacing conventional exploration methods, or post-exploratory, when the instrument is used to check the bile ducts at the conclusion of a conventional exploration. The choledochoscope can also be used post-operatively via the T-tube track to explore and visualize the common and hepatic bile ducts, and to retrieve retained stones (Chapter 7). There are two basic types of choledochoscope, rigid and flexible. The detailed specifications, and techniques associated with each of these, will be considered below.

Conventional methods of surgical exploration of the bile duct for gall-stones are blind techniques dependent only on the surgeon's tactile sense. Any post-exploratory check is confined to an on-table T-tube cholangiogram, which, because of difficulties in performance and interpretation, is often omitted. The incidence of post-operative retained bile duct stones consequently remains unacceptably high.[1-5] The choledochoscope provides the surgeon with a means of exploring the duct under direct vision, facilitating the identification and location of stones. The stones may then be retrieved under direct vision, and a visual post-exploratory check performed so that the incidence of retained stones may be reduced. Indeed, in some cases, the duct may safely be closed primarily without a T-tube drain.

The indications for operative choledochoscopy are the same as those for choledochotomy and exploration: a history of obstructive jaundice, cholangitis, or pancreatitis, with pre-operative investigations suggesting the presence of gall-stones in the common or hepatic bile ducts, palpable common duct stones, or an operative cholangiogram demonstrating a filling defect or obstruction to flow. With a positive pre-operative investigation, it is debatable whether operative cholangiography is necessary and it might be omitted if the surgeon proceeds directly to choledochotomy and exploration of the ducts with a choledochoscope. Once the technique is mastered choledochoscopy is quicker, easier, and more reliable than cholangiography.

HISTORY

Although Thornton inspected the lower end of a much-dilated common bile duct before 1900,[6] the first purpose-built choledochoscope must be attributed to Bakes,[7] who described a speculum with a proximal mirror using reflected light from a surgeon's headlamp; however, this instrument was not developed. The first optical choledochoscope was described by MacIver in 1941, and was produced by A.C.M.I.[8] It was a rigid instrument resembling a cystoscope, with a right-angle 7 cm from the tip, provided with an irrigation channel and a source of light.[9] In 1953, Wildegans of Berlin described a choledochoscope with an optical system enclosed in a rubber sheath, also providing light and irrigation.[10] This was a rigid instrument with a 120°-angle 7 cm from the tip, manufactured by Sass Wolfe & Co., and was developed over several years by Wildegans. He described its use in over 200 cases with only one missed stone.[11] This instrument was developed and adopted by a number of surgeons in the United States, Europe, Scandinavia and Australia.[12-20] Schein described in detail the technique of operative choledochoscopy,[21] and later reported a series of over 100 cases using this instrument.[22] The Storz Company redeveloped the rigid choledochoscope incorporating the Hopkin's rod lens system, giving a much improved optical performance.[23]

The development of fibre-optic endoscopes for use in the gastro-intestinal tract was then extended to choledochoscopy, and the first flexible fibre-optic choledochoscope was described in 1965, manufactured by A.C.M.I.[25] The first British report of the use of this instrument was by Longland.[26] In 1970, the Olympus Optical Company introduced the CHF Series of choledochoscopes with improved fibre-optics and manoeuvrability. During the last decade, other endoscope manufacturers have also produced purpose-built choledochoscopes, and development has continued so that there are now several flexible fibre-optic choledochoscopes fully conforming to the specifications set out later in this chapter. A more detailed history of the development of the choledochoscope is given by Ashby.[27]

THE FLEXIBLE CHOLEDOCHOSCOPE

Several manufacturers include a flexible fibre-optic choledochoscope in their range of endoscopes. A list of those currently available with the salient features and prices of each [at the time of going to press] are shown in Table 4.1. Some of these are designed for multiple use, including bronchos-

Table 4.1

Flexible choledochoscopes.

Make	Model no.	Flexible length (mm)	Tip diameter (mm)	Irrigation channel (mm)	Tip angulation (in one plane)	Optical field (in air)	Basic cost[a] (£)
A.C.M.I.	ACD 15	150	5.0	1.6	220°	70°	3150
A.C.M.I.	ACD 31	310	5.0	1.6	220°	70°	3560
Fujinon	CHS-S	300	6.4	2.6	200°	105°	4100
Olympus	CHF.B3R	280	6.5	2.6	200°	85°	5337
	CHF.4B	330	4.8	2.0	250°	85°	5792
Storz	11001D	330	5.0	2.0	210°	70°	2980
Wolf–Machida	7350	400	5.0	1.6	200°	60°	5353
	7361	400	6.0	2.6	200°	60°	5353
	7370	400	7.0	2.6	200°	60°	5353

[a]U.K. prices in January 1984; all accessories are included in the basic cost.

copy, cystoscopy, and nephroscopy. Because of their flexible construction and fibre-optic light and image-conducting systems, choledochoscopes of this type are naturally more expensive than the rigid instruments. Other considerations, however, enter into the choice of which choledochoscope should be used, besides cost. A comparison of the advantages and disadvantages of the rigid and flexible instruments is made later in this chapter.

Specification requirements

The instrument must be light and well balanced when held in one hand. The flexible working length should be no more than 28–30 cm; greater length may lead to kinking and torsion of the instrument in use, causing loss of control. There should be angulation of the tip of the instrument in one plane, controlled by a simple lever action rather than a wheel or knob; it is essential that the instrument can be manipulated in one hand, leaving the other hand free to manoeuvre the instrument in the bile ducts, or pass accessory devices along the irrigation channel. Angulation in two planes is not necessary as the instrument can be rotated within the duct to vary the plane of angulation.

The diameter of the working length should be as small as possible to facilitate passage of the choledochoscope within the common and hepatic bile ducts. However, an irrigation channel is necessary because choledochoscopy is carried out under continuous fluid irrigation. The diameter of this channel should be as large as possible, commensurate with the diameter of the scope as a whole, because the same channel serves for the passage of accessory devices for engaging with stones under direct vision. This channel should not be less than 2 mm internal diameter. A valve mechanism is necessary at the upper end of the channel so that irrigation is continuous even when a device is being passed down the channel. This valve should be about half-way down the instrument, well away from the operator's face.

THE RIGID CHOLEDOCHOSCOPE

Rigid choledochoscopes are available from two manufacturers. The principle features and prices of each are shown in Table 4.2. Rigid choledochoscopes can also be used for nephroscopy during ureteric exploration.

Specification requirements

The instrument should be light in weight and well balanced. The viewing limb is ideally at right angles to the main shaft. If the angulation is more (e.g. 120°) problems can arise with the shaft coming into contact with the costal

Table 4.2

Rigid choledochoscopes.

Make	Model no.	Working length (mm)	Tip diameter (mm)	Angulation to shaft	Optical field (in air)	Basic cost[a] (£)	Accessories ex VAT (£)
Storz	28022A	60	5.3[b]	90°	80°	739	244
Wolf	8966.31	70	3.7[c]	90°	60°	996	281
Wolf	8967.31	70	5.0[b]	90°	60°	996	281
Wolf	8957.31	70	3.7[c]	120°	60°	949	281
Wolf	8958.31	70	5.0[b]	120°	60°	949	281

[a]U.K. prices in January 1984.
[b]Attachment of the instrument channel increases the diameter to 6.3 mm.
[c]Attachment of the instrument channel increases the diameter to 5.0 mm.

margin before the viewing limb is a sufficient distance into the distal common bile duct.[28] The viewing limb should be 60–70 mm in length. A shorter limb will not always reach the papilla, and a longer limb will sometimes be difficult to insert. The irrigation channel only needs to be large enough for an adequate flow of saline as it is not used for stone retrieval devices. The instrument should be as robust as possible and have entirely waterproof optics. Rigid choledochoscopes have a separate instrument guide which should be simple to attach to the choledochoscope shaft and increase the diameter of the working limb as little as possible. The upper end of this instrument channel should be half-way down the shaft so that instruments can be introduced well away from the operator's face.

STERILIZATION

The choledochoscope is used by the surgeon in the sterile operative field and it is therefore necessary that it should be sterilized. It is not possible, however, to boil or autoclave fibre-optic equipment as it would become irreparably damaged. Most flexible fibre-optic choledochoscopes are now constructed in such a manner that they are entirely waterproof and may be sterilized by total immersion in a chemical agent such as activated glutaraldehyde. Rigid choledochoscopes may be sterilized by total immersion in glutaraldehyde or by low-pressure autoclaving.

An alternative and convenient method of sterilization is by ethylene oxide gas. This has the advantage that the instrument can be maintained in a sterile package on the shelf ready for immediate use, but the disadvantage is that the process takes 36 hours. If the instrument is required for rapid re-use, then it may be sterilized by immersion in glutaraldehyde. It is, of course, essential that the instrument is efficiently cleaned of blood and debris inside as well as outside, immediately after use, and before re-sterilization by either method.

OPERATIVE TECHNIQUE

There are as many variations in minutiae of surgical technique as there are surgeons. However, some details of technique are set out here which the authors have found helpful in facilitating exploration of the common bile duct using both flexible and rigid fibre-optic choledochoscopes.

Although a choledochoscope can be introduced into the common duct regardless of which abdominal incision is used, a transverse right upper abdominal incision is recommended as it affords the best access to the biliary tract when using a choledochoscope. Positioning the patient on the operating table with a modest degree of anti-Trendelenburg and a few degrees of rotation towards the surgeon, who stands on the right of the patient, also improves the general exposure of the biliary tract. The incision should be 2–4 cm above the umbilicus extending to the right just short of the costal margin, and to the left 2 cm across the mid-line. Through this incision the rectus sheath and the rectus muscle are transected with diathermy, and the linea alba divided in the mid-line.[29] The incision should not be extended too far laterally or there is a risk of both damaging segmental nerves and the subsequent development of an incisional hernia. Abdominal packs are inserted over the hepatic flexure of the colon and duodenum, and downward traction is exerted by the assistant's left hand on the structures in the free edge of the lesser omentum. A further retractor is placed beneath the liver to complete the exposure.

Cholecystectomy is carried out and the decision to open and explore the common bile duct is made on the usual indications. The duct is exposed cleanly in its supraduodenal portion and two stay sutures are placed in the duct close to the superior edge of the duodenum. The common duct is opened between these stay sutures and a sample of bile is taken for bacteriological investigation.

Post-exploratory choledochoscopy

When conventional exploration of the common bile duct has been completed, the choledochoscope is used for a post-exploratory visual check. The instrument is introduced into the duct in a distal direction, and the stay sutures crossed over the shaft of the instrument to reduce the leakage of irrigation fluid around the choledochoscope. The irrigation fluid should be warmed, normal saline with a head of pressure of one metre; this flushes bile from the ducts and ensures good choledochoscopic views. Insufficient irrigation pressure allows the unsupported extra hepatic ducts to collapse on to the end of the instrument obscuring the view. The inexperienced choledochoscopist frequently finds difficulty in obtaining adequate views of the distal common bile duct. The choledochoscope is held conveniently in the left hand with the left thumb controlling the angulation lever. The flexible shaft of the choledochoscope in the operative field is best manipulated by means of a pair of long, non-toothed dissecting forceps with rubber pads on the limbs. This enables the operator to manipulate the instrument directly in the common duct. It is not necessary to perform Kocker's mobilization of the second part of the duodenum, nor to insert an assistant's finger behind the common duct during fibre-optic choledochoscopy. When the distal common bile duct has been examined, the instrument is withdrawn from the duct and re-inserted in a proximal direction in order to examine the common hepatic duct and the primary and secondary intrahepatic ducts. This part of the examination is easier because the ducts are supported by the liver tissue and are less likely to impinge on the viewing end of the choledochoscope. In obstructive jaundice with widely dilated ducts it is possible to pass the instrument far up into the tertiary hepatic ducts, 7 or 8 cm into the liver. The carina between the left and right main hepatic ducts must be recognized, and both left and right hepatic duct systems inspected separately. If any residual stones are located by this post-exploratory choledochoscopy, the instrument is removed from the ducts and the ducts re-explored in the conventional manner, since the location of the stone is known. The duct should then be further examined with the choledochoscope before closure. The sequence of proceeding with the examination of the ducts described here is not obligatory. It is immaterial whether the choledochoscope is passed in a proximal or distal direction first, so long as the operator adheres to a routine pattern so that no part of the examination is inadvertently omitted.

Exploratory choledochoscopy

Once the technique of operative, flexible fibre-optic choledochoscopy as a post-exploratory visual check has been mastered, it is but a small step to use the choledochoscope as the exploring instrument, replacing blind conventional techniques with visual exploration of the common bile duct. When the bile duct has been opened, any obvious stones are removed, and the choledochoscope is then introduced into the duct and the exploration carried out under direct vision.

If a gall-stone is located in the bile duct, one of several devices may be passed down the instrument through the valve at the upper end of the

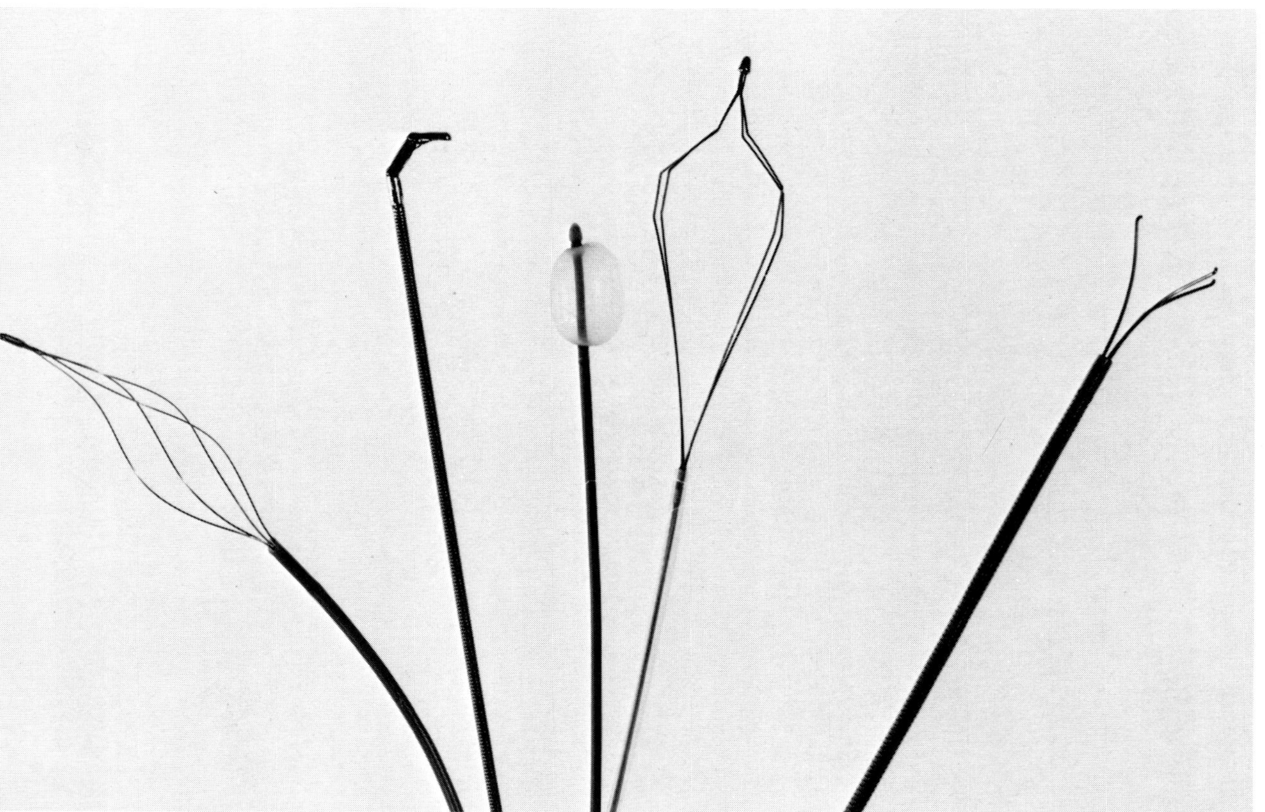

Fig. 4.1 Instruments for use with a choledochoscope. *left to right:* Dormia basket, double-jointed curette, balloon catheter, quadrangular basket, and grasping forceps.

channel while the irrigation continues. Devices available include a Fogarty-type balloon catheter, a wire basket which is particularly useful for the removal of multiple mobile stones within the duct, and a double-jointed curette which can be insinuated beyond a large stone adherent to the duct wall to detach the stone so that it may then be removed (Fig. 4.1). Retrieval of bile duct stones under direct vision in this manner minimizes the trauma inflicted upon the bile duct.

The papilla

When the choledochoscopist is satisfied that all stones and debris have been removed from the common bile duct, and that the hepatic ducts are clear, it is necessary to be sure that the papilla is clear and patent. It is important to be able to recognize the papilla from above. The normal papilla has a rosette appearance. In most cases the flow of irrigation fluid, with the stay sutures crossed to provide a reasonable seal around the endoscope, will indicate that fluid is flowing through the papilla into the duodenum. The papilla may be observed opening and closing as the irrigation fluid passes into the duodenum. If the surgeon is still not satisfied, a balloon catheter may be passed under direct vision through the papilla to demonstrate its patency, and if required, the balloon may be partially inflated within the papilla in order to dilate it. If there is difficulty in recognizing when the choledochoscope has reached the papilla, the balloon catheter is passed through the papilla, the balloon inflated, and the 5 cm gradation mark on the catheter identified choledochoscopically.[30] The catheter is then slowly withdrawn, counting the centimetre marks on it as they pass the viewing lens into the instrument channel, until the 1 cm mark is reached (Fig. 4.2). The choledochoscopist will then be viewing the papilla. Frequently the papilla relaxes sufficiently to obtain a view through into the duodenum. When the surgeon has visually confirmed that all stones and debris have been removed, that the common duct and the hepatic ducts are completely clear, and that the papilla is patent, the procedure is complete.

Rigid choledochoscope — additional points

It is important when using the rigid choledochoscope that the choledocholithotomy incision is low down the common bile duct, just above the upper border of the duodenum. This aids access when the choledochoscope is passed distally, as the shaft of the instrument tends to come up against the costal margin. It is particularly important if an instrument with a working limb angled at 120° is used, but is still advisable with the 90° instrument (Fig. 4.3). In addition, a low incision facilitates choledochoduodenostomy

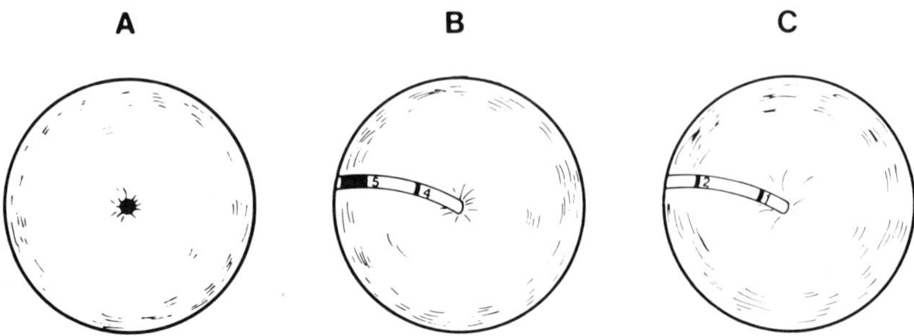

Fig. 4.2 Confirming the papilla has been reached. When the choledochoscopist is uncertain that the papilla has been reached when viewing the distal common bile duct (A) a calibrated balloon catheter is advanced into the duodenum (B). The balloon is inflated and the catheter is then drawn back until the 1 cm mark is in view (C). This confirms that the tip of the endoscope has reached the papilla.

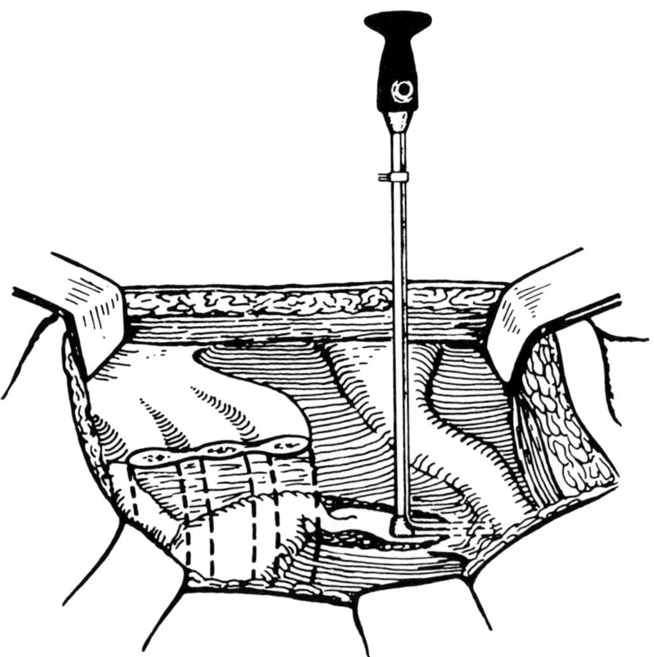

Fig. 4.3 Choledochoscopy with the rigid choledochoscope. The choledochotomy incision is made low down the common bile duct just above the upper border of the duodenum. This keeps the rigid shaft of the choledochoscope away from the costal margin.

should this be necessary. Stay sutures are crossed over the choledochoscope to minimize leakage of the irrigation fluid, as with the flexible instrument. The examination of the proximal ducts is easier, and uniformly good views are obtained. The instrument is then removed, turned through 180°, and introduced into the distal common bile duct. This is undoubtedly the more difficult part of the examination, and attention to detail will ensure a good view. As with flexible choledochoscopy, it does not matter whether the proximal or distal duct is examined first. Good distension of the duct is essential and the infusion should be 1–1.3 metres above the patient to give an adequate head of pressure. If the duct is not adequately distended a uniform red blur is seen on attempted viewing. Division of the peritoneum along the lateral side of the duodenum (Kocker's manoeuvre), mobilizing the head of the pancreas, aids the passage of the rigid instrument to the papilla. With the narrow-gauge Storz or Wolf choledochoscopes, the duodenum can often be entered. This does not occur so frequently with the larger of the Wolf instruments. When the instrument does not pass through one must be quite certain that the tip of the instrument has actually reached the lower end of the duct. A balloon catheter may be used to confirm that the tip of the choledochoscope has reached the papilla, as described above for the flexible instrument (Fig. 4.2).

The rigid choledochoscope may be used either for exploratory or post-exploratory choledochoscopy, as described for the flexible instrument. Stone retrieval can be performed under direct vision by the attachment of an extra channel to the shaft of the instrument to accommodate forceps or balloon catheters, though this does make it a little more cumbersome.[31–33]

Drainage of the common bile duct

When exploration of the bile ducts using choledochoscopy is completed, the question of drainage of the common bile duct arises. A T-tube drain is commonly employed. This is based on a number of factors in conventional exploration — not knowing whether the stones have been completely removed or whether the papilla is really patent, fear of having damaged the ducts during blind exploration, and the possibility of oedema at the lower end of the duct obstructing outflow. A T-tube drain also enables a subsequent post-operative cholangiogram to be performed a week later to confirm that the duct is clear — though any information this provides will be a week too late.

Using choledochoscopy in the manner described, an experienced choledo-choscopist may be satisfied from his visual examination of the ducts, that all stones have been removed, that there is no residual debris, that the common duct and hepatic ducts are clear, and that the papilla is patent. Under these conditions it may be a reasonable course of action to close the common bile duct primarily with no T-tube drain. A continuous 3-0 chromic catgut or polyglycolic acid suture should be used to close the common bile duct, with a corrugated plastic or tubular drain to the subhepatic space in the usual manner.

RESULTS

There is now a considerable reported experience of choledochoscopy, and very satisfactory results are appearing with increasing frequency. Improvements in both the rigid and, in particular, the flexible instruments have accelerated the adoption of the technique. The most recent choledochoscopes on the market are very close to the ideal specifications described above. During the past five years, choledochoscopy has advanced from being a procedure employed primarily by interested enthusiasts to an accepted surgical technique used by more and more surgeons.[34–41] Furthermore, the extensive literature on the treatment of retained stones in recent years has focused attention on the inadequacies of conventional common duct exploration without post-exploratory examination to exclude retained stones.

Does the use of a choledochoscope eliminate retained stones? There are only five reported series with no retained stones at all.[42–46] Two of these were from surgeons using rigid choledochoscopes, and three who used flexible instruments. The overall incidence is low: the mean incidence from 3159 cases collected from the literature is 3.1% (Tables 4.3 and 4.4). In some of these reports the authors have incorrectly related the numbers of retained stones to the total number of choledochoscopies performed (including explorations at which no stones were found) when calculating their percentage incidence of retained stones. This can be very misleading, particularly when there is a high, negative exploration rate. The percentage incidence of retained stones in Tables 4.3 and 4.4 has therefore been related to the number of stone-positive explorations at which the choledochoscope was used. In addition, patients in whom an internal drainage procedure, such as choledochoduodenostomy without T-tube drainage, has been performed, and who therefore lack post-operative confirmation of the presence or absence of stones, have also been omitted. In some cases, therefore, the percentage incidence of retained stones given in the tables is higher than quoted in the original papers. However, even with these exclusions, the mean incidence of 3.1%, although less than ideal, is better than the great majority of reports on conventional exploration even with post-exploratory cholangiography. In only five of the 37 series reported was the incidence greater than 5%, which many surgeons would regard as an acceptable level.[5,61,65,67,73] In

Table 4.3

Flexible choledochoscopy results.

Authors	Year	Stone +ve exploration	No. of retained stones	Percentage of retained stones
Shore and Shore[47]	1970	100	4	4.0
Longland[48]	1975	49	2	4.1
Stotter et al.[43]	1975	20	0	0.0
Finnis and Rowntree[45]	1977	70	0[b]	0.0
Legrand et al.[49]	1978	200	4	2.0
Yap et al.[50]	1980	84	4	4.8
Bauer et al.[51]	1981	36	1	2.8
Grange and Maillard[46]	1981	47	0	0.0
Wang[52]	1982	47	1	2.1
Chen et al.[53]	1982	184	2	1.1
Jakimowicz[54]	1983	115	2	1.7
Jakimowicz et al.[55]	1983	123	3	2.4
Gartell and McGinn[56]	1984	31	1[c]	3.2
Leggeri et al.[57]	1984	128	2	1.6
Ashby	1984	65	1	1.5
TOTAL		1287	27	2.1

[a]Excluding patients having choledochoduodenostomy or other internal drainage and no post-operative T-tube cholangiogam.
[b]Excludes two intrahepatic stones detected but not removed.
[c]Excludes one intrahepatic stone detected but not removed. The retained stone was detected on ERCP 2 years post-operatively.

one of these high incidence reports, 73 choledochoscopies were performed by 13 different surgeons; on average, each will have performed only 5.6 choledochoscopies and this limited experience for some or all of the surgeons may well have contributed to their high rate of stones retained.[61] The results of several of the series of choledochoscopies are comparable to the best that has been achieved by post-exploratory cholangiography. Le Quesne and co-workers achieved excellent results with cholangiography with an incidence of one retained stone in 78 patients (1.3%), but their experience has not been updated since 1975.[74] Others have been unable to match this and most reports quote a 5–10% incidence of retained stones following post-exploratory cholangiography.[75,76]

Although a number of stones which have been missed at choledochoscopy are high in the intrahepatic ducts or, more rarely, are in a cystic duct stump,

Table 4.4

Rigid choledochoscopy results.

Authors	Year	Stone +ve exploration	No. of retained stones	Percentage of retained stones
Wildegans[11]	1958	94	1	1.1
Schein[22]	1969	117	1	0.9
Leslie[42]	1974	71[b]	0	0.0
Shore et al.[58]	1975	70	3	4.3
Griffin[44]	1976	25	0	0.0
Nora et al.[59]	1977	208	4	1.9
Fourtanier et al.[60]	1978	60	1	1.6
Kappas et al.[61]	1979	67	9	13.4
Botticher and Knoch[62]	1980	76	1	1.3
Boulenger et al.[63]	1980	78	1	1.3
Motson et al.[28]	1980	40	2	5.0
Lennert[64]	1980	148	3	2.0
Feliciano et al.[65]	1980	79	7	8.9
Rattner and Warshaw[66]	1980	144	6	4.2
Broadie et al.[67]	1981	32	2	6.3
Ernst and Windsor[68]	1982	38	1	2.7
Kappes et al.[69]	1982	87	2	2.3
Pot[70]	1982	200	9	4.5
Heuman et al.[5]	1982	73	7	9.6
Broe et al.[71]	1983	88	4	3.5
King and String[72]	1983	24	1	4.2
Dayton et al.[73]	1984	53	7[c]	13.2
TOTAL		1872	72	3.8

[a]Excluding patients having choledochoduodenostomy or other internal drainage and no post-operative T-tube cholangiogram.
[b]Includes a few flexible choledochoscopies, majority with rigid choledochoscope.
[c]Excludes one intrahepatic stone detected but not removed.

the great majority of retained stones are left at the lower end of the common bile duct. This must mean that, in these cases, surgeons have mistakenly thought they had reached the lower end of the common duct when they had not actually done so. It is clearly important that a surgeon using the choledochoscope has a clear mental image of the appearances of papilla, and furthermore, they must be certain that he has definitely reached the lower end of the common duct in every case.

Complications

It is difficult to be certain whether complications such as pancreatitis, bile leak from the choledochotomy, or wound infection are attributable to the use of the choledochoscope, as these complications also occur following conventional exploration alone. Certainly, these complications do not seem to be more frequent.[28,45,51,67,73] Kappas, Keighley, and co-workers had one case of septicaemia — a patient with infected bile in whom high infusion pressures were used to clear the duct of debris before choledochoscopy.[61] Recovery was uneventful on a conservative regimen. Injury to the common bile duct is very uncommon. A single case of perforation has occurred while using an older rigid choledochoscope with a 120° rather than 90° viewing limb.[28] This was noted and repaired at the time without further complications. There have been no reports of injuries occurring with either the more modern 90° rigid or the flexible choledochoscopes. There have been two reports of aspiration of infused saline from the nasopharynx when large volumes of irrigation have been used, some of which has refluxed through the pylorus.[77,78] Neither of us has encountered this problem. The technique must now be regarded as very safe with no increase in general or specific complications. Most authors agree that, with experience, it should be possible to achieve the ideal state in which no stones at all are retained.

In almost every series the choledochoscope detected unsuspected stones, or stone fragments, and aided their retrieval either under direct vision or by further instrumentation of the common duct. The number of stones detected varies and is related to the number of stones present, and how assiduous the instrumental exploration has been. One might infer that surgeons who find large numbers of stones with the choledochoscope which were overlooked (e.g. Feliciano, 14%;[65] Motson, 15%;[28] Kappas, 18%;[61] Bauer, 18%;[51] Shore, 22%;[28] Finnis, 27%;[45]) would have had an unacceptably high incidence of retained stones post-operatively if the choledochoscope had not been used. This is because surgeons do not persist with blind instrumentation for very long when a choledochoscope is available, and this will minimize trauma to the bile duct mucosa. The great advantage over cholangiography is the rapidity with which the duct can be examined and, of course, this can be done repeatedly when multiple stones are present without delays for further radiography. In some series[22,59,61] post-exploratory cholangiography has been used as a final check on the choledochoscopic findings. This has identified further stones in a few patients but, as might be expected, the yield has not been high. Once a surgeon is confident in the use of a choledochoscope, and particularly in his interpretation of the appearances of the distal common bile duct and the papilla, it is reasonable to abandon post-exploratory cholangiography.

Choledochoscopy is also valuable in patients without gall-stones. Filling defects such as polyps may be visualized and biopsied. Assessment of strictures both benign and malignant can be assisted by choledochoscopy.[79,80] Although choledochoscopy was devised as an adjunct to supraduodenal exploration of the bile duct, it should not be forgotten when a transduodenal approach has been chosen. Very good views are achieved as one is only viewing in the easier upward direction. The long, flexible choledochoscopes still reach the higher hepatic radicals when used transduodenally, but in some cases rigid choledochoscopes with their fixed-length viewing limb do not visualize beyond the junction of the right and left hepatic ducts.

WHICH CHOLEDOCHOSCOPE?

The following factors are the main things to consider when choosing a choledochoscope.

1. *Facility and versatility.* The ease with which a surgeon becomes accustomed to using a choledochoscope will depend upon existing skills. If used to handling a cystoscope, then a surgeon will at first be more at ease with a rigid choledochoscope. If a surgeon is experienced in fibre-optic endoscopy, then handling a flexible choledochoscope will present no difficulty. There are variations amongst the flexible instruments available and the potential user must feel "comfortable" with an instrument. In the authors' opinion, for example, the angulation control should be a lever action, to facilitate using the choledochoscope in one hand. The manoeuvrability of a rigid scope in a difficult situation may be limited, particularly by the shaft of the instrument fouling the costal margin, whereas a flexible choledochoscope may prove more versatile when the operation is difficult or the patient obese. Accessories attach to the exterior of a rigid choledochoscope, making it a little more cumbersome when they are used.

2. *Optical performance.* With the excellent new generation of fibre-optic bundles now being used in flexible choledochoscopes, and the equally excellent Hopkin's rod lens system in the rigid instrument, there is little to choose between them on optical grounds.

3. *Robustness.* Both types of instrument, of course, need care in cleaning, storing, and sterilizing. There is no evidence that modern fibre-optic choledochoscopes are any more prone to damage, if properly cared for, than their rigid counterparts. Neither is there any indication for limiting the use of a fibre-optic choledochoscope to a few surgeons. It is more important that a fully trained nurse or technician is in charge of the choledochoscope to collect it from the theatre immediately after use, and to clean it and care for it properly.

4. *Sterlization*. Both types of instrument are prepared for use with equal ease, now that most flexible choledochoscopes are totally immersible.

5. *Effectiveness*. On the published evidence reviewed elsewhere in this chapter, the flexible choledochoscope appears to be a little more effective than the rigid choledochoscope in avoiding retained common duct stones.

6. *Cost*. There is a major difference in cost between rigid and flexible choledochoscopes. (The comparative prices of the various instruments are set out in Tables 4.1 and 4.2.) For this reason, many surgeons start choledochoscopy with a rigid instrument, but once they become skilled in the use of the instrument, and are convinced of the value and ease of the procedure, they progress to a flexible fibre-optic choledochoscope.

In summary the flexible choledochoscope is more versatile and may be more difficult to use initially. It is much more costly to purchase or repair if damaged.

THE FUTURE

The trend towards wide acceptance of choledochoscopy will continue as more surgeons try the technique and realize its value. Future development is likely to be in the field of flexible instruments. There are two particular developments of fibre-optic instruments which might usefully be applied to the choledochoscope. One is a totally immersible endoscope, including the light guide and connector, and there is thus no need for watertight sealing caps to be placed over vulnerable parts, making sterilization by immersion even easier. The possibility of a low-temperature steam autoclavable choledochoscope, already achieved with rigid instruments, is attractive but would be rather more difficult with fibre-optic instruments. However, the manufacturers should continue to investigate this as there is a great difference between disinfecting an endoscope adequately for upper gastro-intestinal endoscopy, and sterilizing it for use by the surgeon in a sterile operating field.

The other area for development is reduction in size. Fibre-optic choledochoscopes less than 2 mm in diameter have been evaluated (Fig. 4.4). The difficulty with such instruments is that there is insufficient space to accommodate an irrigation channel and angulation wires, as well as the fibre bundles, and the irrigation channel becomes so small as to affect flow. However, there would be advantages in a choledochoscope that could be pushed through either a large cystic duct or a needle hole in the common bile duct to inspect its interior. Choledochoscopy might then become a routine part of every biliary operation, replacing on-table radiology.

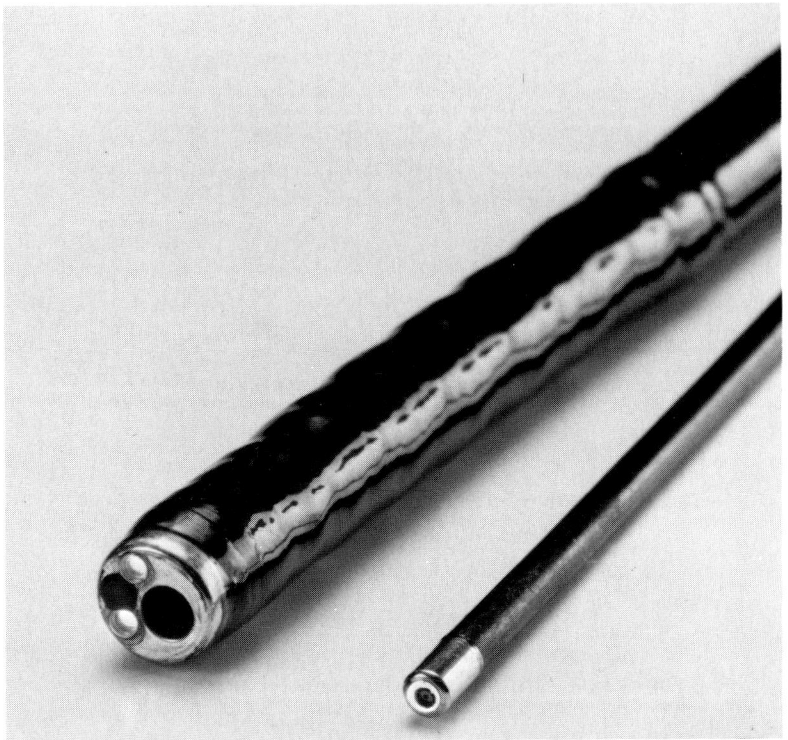

Fig. 4.4 A prototype viewing-only choledochoscope 2 mm in diameter is shown alongside an Olympus CHF-B3 choledochoscope 6.5 mm in diameter.

REFERENCES

1. Hall RC, Sakiyalak P, Kim SK et al. Failure of operative cholangiography to prevent retained common duct stones. Amer J Surg 125: 51–63, 1973.
2. Zimmermann-Nielsen C, Dyreborg U, Madsen CM. Evaluation of peroperative cholangiography during cholecystectomy. Acta Chir Scand 141: 526–531, 1975.
3. Cranley B, Logan H. Exploration of the common bile duct — the relevance of the clinical picture and the importance of peroperative cholangiography. Brit J Surg 67: 869–872, 1980.
4. Reasbeck PG. The results of cholecystectomy at a district general hospital. A reappraisal of operative cholangiography. Ann R Coll Surg Eng 63: 359–362, 1981.
5. Heuman R, Smeds S, Hellgren E et al. Evaluation of factors affecting the incidence of retained calculi in the bile ducts. Acta Chir Scand 145: 185–187, 1982.
6. Madden JL, McCann WJ, Kandalaft S et al. Considerations in surgery of the common duct. Current Problems in Surgery, Chicago, Year Book Medical Publishers, pp. 13–31, 1968.

7.   Bakes J. Die Choledochopapilloskopie hebst bemerkungen uder hepaticus-drainage und dilatation der papille. Arch Klin Chir 126: 473–483, 1923.

8.   McIver MA. An instrument for visualizing the interior of the common duct at operation. Preliminary note. Surgery 9: 112–114, 1941.

9.   McIver MA. Further experience with an instrument for visualising the interior of the common duct at operation. Amer J Dig Dis 9: 52–55, 1942.

10.   Wildegans H. Endoskopie der tiefen gallenwege. Arch Klin Chir 276: 652–659, 1953.

11.   Wildegans H. Endoscopy of the biliary tract. German Med Monthly 3: 377–380, 1958.

12.   Shore JM, Lippman HN. Operative endoscopy of the biliary tract. Ann Surg 156: 951–955, 1962.

13.   Guderley H. Erfahrungen mit der tiefen gallenwege. Zent für Chir 83: 263–265, 1958.

14.   Griessmann H. Intraoperative choledochoscopic study. J Int Coll Surg 31: 644–647, 1959.

15.   Jelinek R. Zur pre- und intraoperativen diagnostik der gallenwegserkrankungen unter besonderer keruksichtigung der Choledochoscopie. Chirurg 30: 358–362, 1959.

16.   Brocks H. Choledochoscopy versus cholangiography. Experience of a 12-month trial. Acta Chir Scand 118: 434–438, 1960.

17.   Berci G. Choledochoscopy. Med J Australia 11: 860–862, 1961.

18.   Leslie D. The use of the choledochoscope; or leaving no stone unturned. Med J Australia 1: 235–236, 1962.

19.   Schein CJ, Stern WZ, Jacobson HG. The hepatic ductal system: a correlation of endoscopic and roentgenographic findings. Surgery 51: 718–723, 1962.

20.   Schein CJ, Stern WZ, Hurwitt ES et al. Cholangiography and biliary endoscopy as complementary methods of evaluating the bile ducts. Amer J Roentgenol 89: 864–875, 1963.

21.   Schein CJ, Hurwitt ES. The technique of biliary tract endoscopy. Surg Gynecol Obstet 113: 514–516, 1961.

22.   Schein CJ. Biliary endoscopy: an appraisal of its value in biliary lithiasis. Surgery 65: 1004–1006, 1969.

23.   Shore JM, Morgenstern L, Berci G. An improved rigid choledochoscope. Amer J Surg 122: 567–568, 1971.

24.   Berci G, Shore JM. Advances in cholangioscopy. Endoscopy 4: 29–31, 1972.

25.   Shore JM, Lippman HN. A flexible choledochoscope. Lancet i: 1200–1201, 1965.

26.   Longland CJ. Choledochoscopy in choledocholithiasis. Brit J Surg 60: 626–628, 1973.

27.   Ashby BS. Choledochoscopy. Clin Gastroenterol 7: 685–700, 1978.

28.   Motson RW, Wood AJ, de Jode LR. Operative choledochoscopy: experience with a rigid choledochoscope. Brit J Surg 67: 406–409, 1980.

29.   Ashby B.S. Operative choledochoscopy. Rob and Smith's Operative Surgery, 4th Edn (H Dudley, W Pories and D Carter Eds). Alimentary Tract and Abdominal Wall, Vol 2, Butterworths, London, p. 644, 1983.

30.   Ross H. An aid to the complete visualization of the bile duct with the Storz choledochoscope. Surg Gynecol Obstet 150: 574–575, 1980.

31.   Shore JM, Berci G. Operative management of calculi in the hepatic ducts. Amer J Surg 119: 625–631, 1970.

32. Warshaw AL, Bartlett MK. Technic for finding and removing stones from intrahepatic bile ducts. Amer J Surg 127: 353–354, 1974.
33. Ottinger LW, Warshaw AL, Bartlett MK. Intraoperative endoscopic evaluation of the bile ducts. Amer J Surg 127: 465–468, 1974.
34. Ferry C, Montagnon J, Rollier J et al. Place de la choledocoscopie per-operatoire dans la chirurgie de la lithiase; a propos de 40 cas. Ann Med Reims 12: 9–11, 1975.
35. Vosse A. Aspects endoscopiques per-operatoires des voies biliaires. Acta Endosc 6: 3–7, 1976.
36. Berci G, Shore JM, Morgenstern L et al. Choledochoscopy and operative fluorocholangiography in the prevention of retained bile duct stones. World J Surg 2: 411–427, 1978.
37. Iseli A, Marshall VC. Choledochoscopy: a comparison of a rigid and a flexible fibreoptic instrument. Med J Australia 1: 131–132, 1978.
38. Ashby BS. Fibreoptic choledochoscopy in common bile duct surgery. Ann R Coll Surg Eng 60: 399–403, 1978.
39. Keighley MRB, Kappas A. Evaluation of operative choledochoscopy. Surg Gynecol Obstet 150: 357–359, 1980.
40. Cooperman A, Gelbfish G, Zimmon DS. Choledochoscopy. Surg Clin N Amer 62: 853–859, 1982.
41. Wang Y-H. Choledochoscopy versus cholangiography. SE Asian J Surg 4: 50–57, 1981.
42. Leslie D. Endoscopy of the bile duct: an evaluation. Aust NZ J Surg 44: 340–342, 1974.
43. Stotter L, Wiendl H-J, Ultsch B. An improved flexible cholangioscope. Endoscopy 7: 150–153, 1975.
44. Griffin WT, Choledochoscopy. Amer J Surg 132: 697–698, 1976.
45. Finnis D, Rowntree T. Choledochoscopy in exploration of the common bile duct. Brit J Surg 64: 661–664, 1977.
46. Grange D, Maillard J-N. La choledocoscopie peroperatoire. Gastroenterol Clin Biol 5: 857–865, 1981.
47. Shore JM, Shore E. Operative biliary endoscopy: experience with the flexible choledochoscope in 100 consecutive choledocholithotomies. Ann Surg 171: 269–278, 1970.
48. Longland CJ. Cited by Ashby BS. Choledochoscopy. Clin Gastroenterol 7: 685–700, 1978.
49. Legrand G, Izard G, Cave C et al. La choledocoscopie per-operatoire dans la chirurgie de la lithiase de la voie biliare principale. Á propos de 200 cas. Lyon Chir 74: 321–324, 1978.
50. Yap PC, Atacador M, Yap AG et al. Choledochoscopy as a complementary procedure to operative cholangiography in biliary surgery. Amer J Surg 140: 648–652, 1980.
51. Bauer JJ, Salky BA, Gelernt IM et al. Experience with the flexible fibreoptic choledochoscope. Ann Surg 196: 161–168, 1982.
52. Wang Y-H. The use of operative choledochoscope. J Formosan Med Assoc 81: 1140–1143, 1982.
53. Chen M-F, Jan Y-Y, Chou F-F et al. Use of fibreoptic choledochoscope in common bile duct and intrahepatic duct exploration. Gastrointest Endosc 29: 276–278, 1983.
54. Jakimowicz JJ. Operative choledochoscopy using the flexible choledochoscope,

a six year experience. 30th Congress, International Society of Surgery, Hamburg, 1983.

55. Jakimowicz JJ, Carol EJ, Mak B. Operative choledochoscopy using the flexible choledochoscope, a six year experience. 30th Congress, International Society of Surgery, Hamburg, 1983.

56. Gartell PC, McGinn FP. Choledochoscopy: are stones missed? A prospective controlled study. Brit J Surg 71: 767–769, 1984.

57. Leggeri A, Liguori G, Umeri F. Intraoperative choledochoscopy. Padua, Piccin & Butterworths, pp. 83–88, 1984.

58. Shore JM, Berci G, Morgenstern L. The value of biliary endoscopy. Surg Gynecol Obstet 140: 601–604, 1975.

59. Nora PF, Berci G, Dorazio RA et al. Operative choledochoscopy. Results of a prospective study in several institutions. Amer J Surg 133: 105–110, 1977.

60. Fourtanier G, Lacroix A, Escat J. L'interet de la choledochoscopie au cours de l'exploration de la voie biliare principale pour lithiase. Ann Chir 32: 122–125, 1978.

61. Kappas A, Alexander-Williams J, Keighley MRB et al. Operative choledochoscopy. Brit J Surg 66: 177–179, 1979.

62. Botticher R, Knoch M. Diagnostischer und therapeutischer stellenwert der intraoperativen choledochoskopie. Langenbecks Arch Chir 351: 17–22, 1980.

63. Boulenger M, Solente JJ, Moline J et al. La choledocoscopie per-operatoire. A propose de 120 cas. Lyon Chir 75: 166–167, 1979.

64. Lennert KA. Die intraoperative Choledochoskopie. Erfahrungen mit einem neuen Choledochoskop. Chirurg 47: 248–249, 1976.

65. Feliciano DV, Mattox KL, Jordan GL Jr. The value of choledochoscopy in exploration of the common bile duct. Ann Surg 191: 649–654, 1980.

66. Rattner DW, Warshaw AL. Impact of choledochoscopy on the management of choledocholithiasis. Experience with 499 common duct explorations at the Massachusetts General Hospital. Ann Surg 194: 76–79, 1981.

67. Broadie TA, Lowe DK, Glover JL et al. Intraoperative choledochoscopy: an efficacious adjunct to common duct exploration in calculous biliary tract disease. Am Surg 47: 121–124, 1981.

68. Ernst D, Windsor CWO. The use of a rigid choledochoscope in exploration of the common bile duct. Brit J Surg 69: 463–464, 1982.

69. Kappes SK, Adams MB, Wilson SD. Intraoperative biliary endoscopy. Mandatory for all common duct operations? Arch Surg 117: 603–607, 1982.

70. Pot JH. Peroperative investigation with a rigid choledochoscope. Association of Surgeons, Manchester, 1982.

71. Broe PJ, Magee DJ, Kirwan WO. Value of choledochoscopy in exploration of the common bile duct. Gut 24: 503, 1983.

72. King ML, String ST. Extent of choledochoscopic utilization in common bile duct exploration. Amer J Surg 146: 322–324, 1983.

73. Dayton MT, Conter R, Tompkins RK. Incidence of complications with operative choledochoscopy. Amer J Surg 147: 139–145, 1984.

74. Faris I, Thomson JPS, Grundy DJ et al. Operative cholangiography: a reappraisal based on a review of 400 cholangiograms. Brit J Surg 62: 966–972, 1975.

75. Isaacs JP, Davies ML. Technique and evaluation of operative cholangiography. Surg Gynecol Obstet 111: 103–112, 1960.

76. Way LW, Admirand WH, Dunphy JE. Management of choledocholithiasis. Ann Surg 176: 347–359, 1972.

77. Weller RM. The choledochoscope — two hazards. Anaesthesia 37: 606, 1982.
78. Schebesta AG, Sporr D, O'Leary J et al. Gastric aspiration associated with operative choledochoscopy. Anaes Int Care 11: 257–258, 1983.
79. Tompkins RK, Johnson J, Storm FK et al. Operative endoscopy in the management of biliary tract neoplasms. Amer J Surg 132: 174–182, 1976.
80. Schein CJ. Influence of choledochoscopy on the choice of surgical procedure. Amer J Surg 130: 74–77, 1975.

5

Dissolution and Flushing of Retained Common Bile Duct Stones

Roger W. Motson and Lawrence W. Way

At present, stone extraction techniques, either using the T-tube track or endoscope, have the greatest success in the treatment of common duct stones. However, flushing and dissolution still have an important role, particularly when stone extraction techniques are unavailable or unsuccessful.

There has been considerable interest in dissolution of retained common duct stones during the last decade, but the idea is not new. The first attempts at dissolution took place more than 90 years ago,[1] and many patients have been successfully treated over the years. Optimistic reports in the 1930s led to widespread use of a variety of solvents.[2-7] Unpredictable results, lengthy treatment periods, and the lack of an efficient and reliable solvent contributed to a decline in the use of dissolution, and re-operation remained the principal treatment.

In 1968, Admirand and Small demonstrated that bile from patients with gall-stones was supersaturated with cholesterol, whereas bile from normal subjects was undersaturated.[8] Cholesterol from supersaturated bile precipitated to form cholesterol crystals. Solid cholesterol could be resolubilized by exposure to unsaturated bile. The elucidation of these principles led Way and his colleagues to try physiological concentrations of bile salts free of cholesterol for dissolution of retained gall-stones in the common bile duct.[9] This rekindled interest in dissolution of retained stones and brought about a more thorough examination of potentially effective gall-stone solvents.

The reported results of dissolution therapy for retained gall-stones are somewhat confusing and at times contradictory. Most of the reports are anecdoctal, and there are no adequate controlled trials. The composition of gall-stones determines whether dissolution is possible, and some treatment failures may have resulted from inappropriate selection of patients. Furthermore, sudden disappearance of stones has often been equated with dissolution, even though other explanations are plausible. For example, the irrigating fluid may carry the gall-stone, particularly if it is small, intact into the duodenum; the stone may fragment into pieces individually small enough to pass; or true gall-stone dissolution, sometimes confirmed by decreasing stone diameter on repeated T-tube cholangiography, may occur.

GALL-STONE COMPOSITION

Gall-stones are composed principally of bile pigments, cholesterol, or a mixture of these and other substances. For gall-stone dissolution to be successful the chosen solvent must be capable of dissolving the predominant constituent of the stone. In both the United Kingdom and the United States, cholesterol and mixed cholesterol stones constitute about 75% of gall-stones, and pigment stones the remaining 25%.[10,11] *Pigment stones* are more common in women than men (M:F, 2:3), and are more often found in elderly patients.[12] Haemolytic disease and alcoholic cirrhosis are known aetiologic factors, but they are present in only a minority of patients. Most pigment stones are composed of calcium bilirubinate, bile salts, small amounts of cholesterol, and an insoluble pigment residue (bilirubin polymers) that accounts for two-thirds of the total weight. In vitro studies have shown that ethylene-diamine-tetra-acetic acid (EDTA) can dissolve calcium bilirubinate, the principle component of most pigment stones.[13] After a continuous infusion of EDTA into the common bile ducts of dogs every day for 4 weeks, histological examination showed desquamation of the common bile duct mucosa in three, cellular infiltration of the portal tracts in six, and portal fibrosis in two.[13] Clinical use of EDTA has been reported by Leuschner and colleagues, but their patients also received bile acids and mono-octanoin which makes interpretation of the role of EDTA impossible.[14] In view of the histologic damage in animals, clinical use of EDTA must be very cautious. At present, there is no solvent of proven safety available for pigment stones, and attempts at dissolution must therefore be confined to patients with cholesterol stones.

Cholesterol stones are also more common in women (M:F, 1:4), in middle age, and in the presence of obesity. Cholesterol accounts for 70% or more of the total stone weight, with small amounts of bile salts, and bilirubin. Calcium salts, usually calcium carbonate, are also present, and accounted for 24% of the stone weight in one series.[15] The presence of this insoluble matrix undoubtedly contributes to the variable success achieved with dissolution.

GALL-STONE SOLVENTS

A wide variety of solvents has been tried over the years, but the most successful ones have been ether, chloroform, bile salts, and more recently, mono-octanoin.

Ether

The first report of gall-stone dissolution with ether was in 1891, in a patient who became jaundiced after cholecystostomy as a result of a common bile duct stone. A mixture of ether and glycerine was instilled into the gall bladder through a tube, and two days later the stone could not be felt.[1] This report went largely unnoticed, and it was not until 1935 that the method was revived by Pribram.[16] He performed cholangiography on the fifth day post-operatively, and after aspirating bile, slowly instilled ether into the T-tube until the patient felt pain or pressure, at which point ether was re-aspirated. He repeated the procedure several times a week, sometimes for several weeks, and claimed a 100% success rate in a series of over 50 cases.[16].

The principal difficulty with ether is its low boiling point. At normal body temperature, 1 ml of liquid ether will vaporize to form over 220 ml of gaseous ether, and some of the early reports show considerable gaseous dilatation of bile duct, duodenum, and stomach.[7] Pancreatitis and cholangitis were surprisingly infrequent. Pain occurred in most patients, and attempts were made to alleviate this by using double-lumen tubes to vent the gas, and less volatile mixtures of ether and alcohol.[17,18].

Overall, it seems unlikely that dissolution was common with ether. The rapid vaporization meant that contact between the stone and liquid ether could only have lasted for a few seconds. Furthermore, only pure cholesterol stones are dissolved rapidly by ether, and mixed stones require much longer treatment. In retrospect, the successes were probably achieved more by the ether vapour forcing the stones out of the duct than by true dissolution.

Chloroform

Chloroform, a most efficient cholesterol solvent, dissolves gall-stones in vitro in a few hours. Unfortunately, it has the potential to cause serious side effects when used in vivo. Centrilobular hepatic necrosis and several deaths occurred in animal experiments,[19] and duodenal ulceration and haemorrhage were reported after its use in patients. Nevertheless, chloroform was used successfully by Best and co-workers for over 30 years as part of a regimen of T-tube installations and oral choleretics.[20] The Best regimen never gained widespread use, however, no doubt as a result of both reported and unreported complications.

Bile salts

It has been known since the turn of the century that human gall-stones dissolve when placed in animal bile. In 1932 it was shown that bile salts maintained the cholesterol in solution in bile,[21] and in 1937 Rewbridge used oral bile salts in attempts to dissolve gall-stones in patients with functioning gall bladders.[22] His success went unnoticed, and it is only recently that interest has been renewed in oral bile salt therapy.[23] Early in vitro surveys also investigated bile salts as potential gall-stone solvents when applied directly to retained stones. Only weak (10%) solutions were tested and these were ineffective.[19]

Bile salts hold cholesterol in solution by forming micelles. In aqueous solution the hydrophilic pole of the bile salt is in contact with the surrounding molecules of water and the lipophilic poles face each other. Within the lipid interior of the micelle, cholesterol or other lipids can be dissolved, while the mixture remains in aqueous solution. The phospholipid lecithin increases the size of the micelle, which allows more cholesterol to be held in solution. Cholesterol gall-stones form in bile supersaturated with respect to cholesterol (i.e. there are insufficient micelles available). Cholesterol gall-stones dissolve if exposed to bile salt solutions unsaturated with respect to cholesterol (i.e. there are unsaturated micelles available), and this forms the basis for using bile salts clinically to treat retained common duct stones.

The steps involved in dissolution are: diffusion of micelles to the stone surface; entry of cholesterol molecules into the micelle; and diffusion of the cholesterol-containing micelles away from the stone. When flow is slow or stagnant, diffusion controls the rate of dissolution, but when the rate of flow is fast (as in T-tube infusion), events at the stone surface control the rate of dissolution. In most cases, adsorption of the micelle onto the surface of the gall-stone is the rate-limiting step.[24] The process is relatively straightforward when dealing with pure cholesterol stones (or cholesterol pellets), but is much more complicated when an inert matrix, such as pigment, calcium, etc., acts as a barrier to micellar diffusion.[25,26] This is probably why the results of dissolution therapy are unpredictable.

In vitro studies confirm the efficacy of bile salts as gall-stone solvents. Earnest and Admirand showed sodium deoxycholate to be more effective than either cholate or chenodeoxycholate in stagnant solutions,[27] a finding confirmed by others.[28] However, when the solvent solutions were investigated in a flowing system, more akin to the conditions during clinical use, the differences disappeared[29] (Fig. 5.1). The use of lecithin to increase the size of the micelle might be expected to increase the efficacy of dissolution by allowing more cholesterol to be transported, but in practice lecithin retards dissolution.[30,31] The explanation may be that the increased micellar size interferes with its adsorption to the stone surface. In addition, bigger micelles may diffuse more slowly, particularly when an inert matrix is present.

Additives to the solvent solution alter the rate of dissolution, probably by

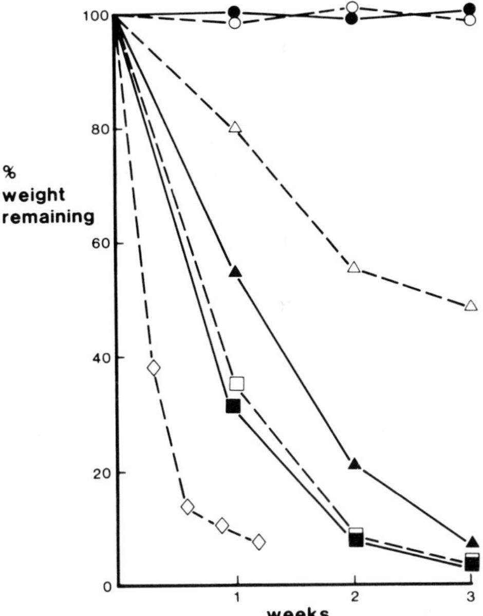

Fig. 5.1 Dissolution of cholesterol gall-stones in vitro. There is no difference between heparin and the saline control. Increasing concentrations of cholic and deoxycholic acid are more efficient, but the most rapid dissolution is achieved by mono-octanoin. ○ 0.15 N NaCl; ● heparin 10,000 U/ml; △ 100 m cholic acid; ▲ 100 m deoxycholic acid; □ 150 m cholic acid; ■ 150 m deoxycholic acid; ◇ mono-octanoin.

affecting adsorption of the micelles. Sodium chloride is the most important. Molokhia and colleagues showed that increasing the sodium chloride concentration without altering the bile salt concentration increases the rate of dissolution considerably.[32] Quaternary amines and heparin, which seem to foster stone fragmentation rather than dissolution, have both been used as additives.[33] However, when added to cholic acid solutions, they have not been found to increase the rate of gall-stone dissolution.[29] Other compounds such as trypsin, papain, pancreatin, and acetylcyteine have all been added to cholate solutions without beneficial effects.[29]

Interest in bile salts was renewed in 1972 by the report from Way, Admirand, and Dunphy, which described successful dissolution of retained common duct stones with cholic acid in 12 (55%) out of 22 patients.[9] They employed 100 mM sodium cholate, infused at a rate of 30 ml/h. The only side-effects were intestinal colic and diarrhoea due to the large volumes of bile salt entering the intestine. This was minimized by giving the patients cholestyramine, a bile salt binding resin. Treatment was time-consuming,

Table 5.1

Dissolution of gall-stones with bile salts.

Authors	Year	No. successful	No. treated	Per cent success
Way et al.[9]	1972	12	22	54.6
Lansford et al.[34]	1974	5	6	83.3
Mok et al.[35]	1974	2	4	50.0
Toouli et al.[36]	1974	13	16	81.3
Britton et al.[37]	1975	4	7	57.1
La Russo et al.[38]	1975	2	6	33.3
Way and Motson[39]	1976	9	14	64.3
Wheeler[40]	1977	2	3	66.6
Christiansen et al.[41]	1978	3	7	42.9
James[42]	1979	7	11	63.6
Sohrabi et al.[43]	1979	6	8	75.0
Motson[44]	1981	5	9	55.6
TOTAL		70	113	61.9

however, usually lasting about two weeks and requiring hospitalization. The success achieved encouraged others to experiment with cholic acid infusions.[34-44] Varying results have been reported, and with our further experience, 70 out of 113 (62%) patients reported have been treated successfully (Table 5.1).

Oral bile salt therapy has been largely directed to treatment of patients with small radiolucent stones in functioning gall bladders, rather than patients with retained common bile duct stones. Nevertheless, there have been a number of case reports of disappearance of common duct stones in response to oral chenodeoxycholic acid.[45,46] Ursodeoxycholic acid has recently been evaluated in a double blind randomized trial in which dissolution was confirmed in 57% patients.[47] The treatment period was intended to be two years, but only four of 28 patients completed the trial, either because the stones had disappeared or because patients left the trial with biliary pain, cholangitis, elective surgery, or simply "dropped out". Symptoms and surgery were all more common in the placebo group. Oral therapy is expensive and slow, and it does not at present compare with the other available techniques.[48]

Heparin

The use of heparin as a gall-stone solvent was advocated by Ostrowitz and Gardner in 1970.[49] They demonstrated in vitro that this highly negatively charged molecule could improve the stability of colloidal suspensions by increasing the surface charge of individual particles. They suggested that micelles in bile salt solutions would behave like colloidal particles, and that heparin should enhance dissolution. Subsequently they reported a successful clinical outcome in 31 (72%) out of 43 patients.[50] Two additional clinical reports have appeared from Gardner[51] and Chary.[52] However, subsequent laboratory studies have cast doubt that heparin possesses any solvent effect. One study has demonstrated fragmentation in vitro using heparin as an additive to sodium cholate,[33] but other workers have failed to show any effect of heparin either alone or in combination with cholate or deoxycholate.[9,39,53-56] A variety of concentrations have been tried without benefit in both stagnant and flowing solvent systems.

These findings suggest that heparin has no direct effect on dissolution of cholesterol gall-stones. It seems likely that the clinical successes achieved were due to simple flushing.

Clofibrate

The use of the hypocholesterolaemic agent clofibrate for gall-stone dissolution was suggested following in vitro studies in which stones dissolved in 2–3 weeks when exposed to a clofibrate–alcohol solution,[57] and successful stone dissolution was reported in one patient.[58] Although this patient's stones disappeared, diminution in stone size was not shown on any of the films. When in vitro studies were repeated using identical solutions, stone softening and fragmentation occurred, but the same effect was seen in an ethyl alcohol control. Overall it seems unlikely that clofibrate is an effective solvent.

Mono-octanoin

Mono-octanoin, a medium chain triglyceride (octanoic acid esterified to glycerol at the α-position), is available commercially as the predominant constituent of Capmul, a capric acid emulsifier, produced by Stokely-Van Camp, Inc. of Indianapolis, U.S.A. Mono-octanoin is a yellow liquid that emulsifies readily with water or bile, and as its freezing point is between room and body temperature, it is often semi-solid when received.

Thistle and co-workers at the Mayo Clinic first reported the results of in vitro studies with mono-octanoin in 1977.[59] Matched pairs of gall-stones were incubated in 150 mM sodium cholate and mono-octanoin solutions. The rate of dissolution was 2.5 times greater in mono-octanoin; findings which were confirmed later by several other groups.[44,60,61].

Animal studies suggested that mono-octanoin was safe for use in man.[62] Following the in vitro reports, clinical use was soon reported, first by Thistle

Table 5.2

Dissolution of gall-stones with mono-octanoin.

Authors	Year	No. successful	No. treated	Per cent success
Thistle et al.[63]	1980	10	12	83.3
Wurbs et al.[64]	1980	6	10	60.0
Schenk et al.[65]	1980	3	5	60.0
Jarrett et al.[66]	1981	15[a]	24	62.5
Mack et al.[67]	1981	15	20	75.0
Uribe et al.[68]	1981	6	12	50.0
Leuschner et al.[14]	1981	12[b]	20	60.0
Gadacz[69]	1981	5	8	62.0
Cassat and Shannon[70]	1982	1	1	100.0
Venu et al.[71]	1982	7	9	77.8
Dawson and Cockel[72]	1982	10[c]	17	58.8
Velasco et al.[73]	1983	13[d]	20	65.0
Motson	1983	3	5	60.0
TOTAL		106	163	65.0

[a]Includes 5 partial successes (decreased size, not completely dissolved).
[b]Includes 4 partial successes (also received bile acids and EDTA).
[c]Includes 1 partial success.
[d]Includes 4 partial successes.

and co-workers at the Mayo Clinic in 1978,[63] and subsequently by others[44, 64–73] (Table 5.2). The success of the Mayo group has not quite been equalled by others, but diminution in size has been shown in serial films, and if partial successes are included, nearly 70% of patients have been treated successfully, a rate similar to that with cholic acid. Although less frequent than with cholic acid, diarrhoea does occur in some patients, and both cholangitis and systemic side-effects have been reported.[73,74]

FLUSHING

Retained stones may also be induced to pass from the bile duct by the hydraulic force of the infusion, particularly when the stone is sited distally. Flushing can be achieved by installing solutions directly into the T-tube or by administering oral choleretics. Best reported an 80% success rate using deoxycholic acid as an oral choleretic, together with oral atropine, magnesium sulphate, and olive oil to relax the sphincter of Oddi.[20] Treatment was often prolonged. Cole and Harridge fed bile salts (principally cholic acid)

Table 5.3

Removal of gall-stones by saline irrigation.

Authors	Year	No. successful	No. treated	Per cent success
Catt et al.[76]	1974	6	10	60.0
Mackie et al.[77]	1975	2	2	100.0
Castelden[78]	1976	4	8	50.0
Motson	1983	7	12	58.3
TOTAL		19	32	59.4

3–4 g/day to nine patients with retained stones, and in seven patients the stones disappeared.[75] Cholic acid is not an effective solvent when used orally, so the success in these patients was probably due to a choleretic action.

Flushing via the T-tube has produced better results than might have been expected (Table 5.3).[44,76-78] Saline has been the most widely used irrigant. It has been given by forceful injection, apparently without causing cholangitis or other ill effects, but most workers attempt to keep pressures within the physiologic range. Topical anaesthetics, nitrates, and anticholinergic drugs have all been added to the flushing solutions in attempts to relax the sphincter of Oddi and ease stone passage.[79,80] None has been used in a systematic way, and it is not possible to determine if these agents have contributed to success. Overall, a successful outcome occurs in about 50% of cases, and flushing is a useful preliminary manoeuvre when a retained stone is first discovered. As well as disposing of some stones, it will also clear the ducts of air bubbles and blood clots, which sometimes simulate stones. Methods that claim successful dissolution without demonstrating decreasing stone size on serial cholangiograms must be viewed against results achieved by non-solvent solutions.

INFUSION TECHNIQUES

T-tube infusion

A standard central venous pressure intravenous giving set is used. The manometer limb is cut short at 30 cm to prevent intrabiliary pressure from rising above this level (Fig. 5.2). The giving set can be coupled directly to the end of the T-tube, but a higher concentration of solvent around the stone can be achieved if a fine catheter is advanced up to the stone under fluoroscopic

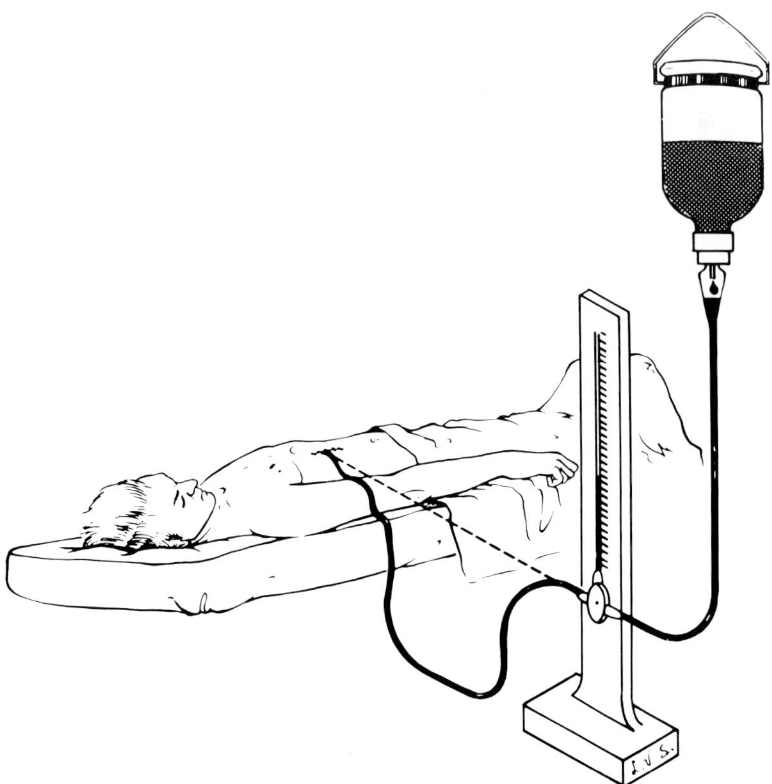

Fig. 5.2 The infusion system. The solvent is administered via an intravenous infusion set with a manometer side arm which is cut short at 30 cm to prevent any higher rises in pressure if the stone should obstruct the bile duct.

control. This technique should always be used if the stone is proximal to the T-tube. It may also be possible to achieve higher concentrations around distally placed stones by using a two-lumen balloon catheter in the distal common duct, which diverts bile out of the T-tube and keeps the solvent in contact with the stone undiluted (Fig. 5.3).

Nasobiliary infusion

Dissolution has been used as an adjunct to endoscopic stone removal when the stones are too large (>2 cm) to pass through the ampulla after sphincterotomy. At the end of the endoscopic procedure a long catheter is passed through the instrument channel of the endoscope, into the open ampulla, and up the bile duct, where several centimetres of catheter are made

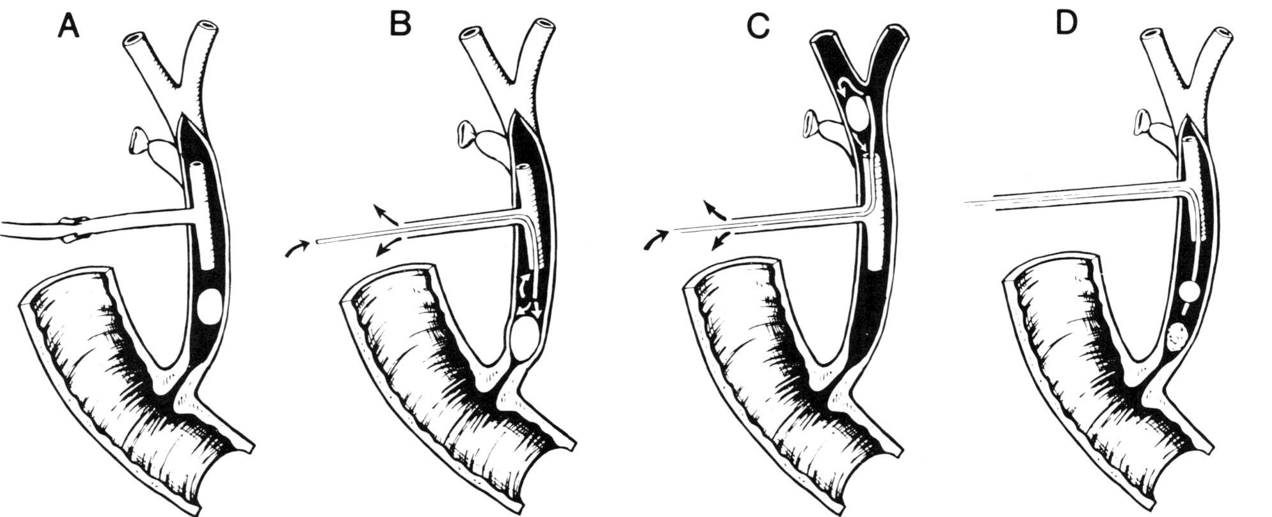

Fig. 5.3   (A) The infusion may be connected directly to the end of the T-tube, provided the stone is not obstructing the duct. (B) If the duct is obstructed, a fine catheter is advanced through the T-tube up to the stone, bile and solvent escape back along the T-tube. (C) If the stone is situated in the proximal ducts a fine catheter is advanced beyond the stone. (D) High concentrations of solvent may be achieved around stones situated distally by using a two-lumen balloon catheter which diverts bile out of the T-tube and keeps the solvent in contact with the stone undiluted by bile.

to curl up above the stone to prevent the catheter from falling out.[81] The endoscope is then removed over the catheter, which is re-routed from the mouth to the nose. Mono-octanoin is infused at a rate of 10 ml/h, which is faster than when given down a T-tube, because the open ampulla allows freer passage from the duct. Early experience has shown that there is sufficient dissolution for these stones to pass through the sphincterotomized ampulla.

Percutaneous transhepatic infusion

The great improvements in transhepatic cholangiography achieved by the use of the Chiba or "skinny" needle, which can cannulate successfully over 60% of non-dilated ducts,[82] has led recently to the use of the transhepatic route for infusing solvents in patients who no longer have T-tubes. After cannulation of the biliary tree, and confirmation of the presence of a retained stone, a catheter is introduced over a guide wire by standard Seldinger technique. Cholangiograms are taken to confirm that the catheter tip is within the hepatic duct before the infusion is started.[83] Mack and colleagues placed a second catheter in the bile ducts when distal obstruction was complete, to vent the obstructed duct and prevent development of high intraduct pressures.[84] However, it is probably equally effective in such circumstances to relieve the obstruction and then aspirate as much bile as possible. If mono-octanoin is then instilled and the patient stood erect, the solvent settles into the distal biliary tree, and the catheter may be used to drain newly formed bile from above the solvent.

CURRENT RECOMMENDATIONS

Retained stones are usually discovered on T-tube cholangiograms 7–10 days post-operatively. The first treatment should probably be irrigation with saline using the T-tube infusion system described above. Although some workers have recommended early use of stone solvents, we prefer to do nothing further at this stage if saline irrigation is unsuccessful. The reasons are twofold: first, some stones pass spontaneously; secondly, the T-tube track must be allowed to heal soundly before solvent solutions are instilled or instruments introduced. During this waiting period, which should be 5–6 weeks, the patient may be discharged home, either with the T-tube spigotted if there is free flow past the stone into the duodenum, or on free drainage if the common duct is completely obstructed by the stone.

If the stone is still present 6 weeks post-operatively, then spontaneous passage is unlikely. The decision to use a gall-stone solvent will to some extent, depend on whether T-tube basket extraction (Chapter 6), choledochoscopic extraction (Chapter 7) or endoscopic extraction (Chapter 8) are available. If all are available, and the T-tube remains in situ, then extraction under radiologic control should be the first choice, since it has a high chance of success ($>90\%$) and a low morbidity. If all are unavailable, then the simple but less efficient technique of gall-stone dissolution may be utilized.

Before attempting stone dissolution it is advisable to test a gall bladder stone in vitro to see if it dissolves in cholesterol solvents. Morphologic studies have shown that 97% of common duct stones have the same composition as the gall bladder stones from the same patient.[84] If dissolution does not occur in vitro it is most unlikely to occur in vivo. The best results have been achieved by groups using mono-octanoin, although the accumulated experience (65.0%, Table 5.2) differs litle from that for cholic acid (61.9%, Table 5.1). Mono-octanoin is infused at a rate of 5 ml/h after sterilization by filtration through a 0.22 μm filter. Cholic acid is a second choice, although in practice it is about as safe and effective as mono-octanoin. A 150 mM solution is used, sterilized either by autoclaving or millipore filtration (0.22 μm filter).

It is probably unreasonable to persist with attempts at dissolution for more than 2–3 weeks without evidence of decreasing stone size. At this point the patient should be referred to a centre where stone extraction techniques are available.

REFERENCES

1. Walker JW. The removal of gallstones by ether solution. Lancet i: 874–875, 1891.
2. Pribram BO. New methods in gallstone surgery. Surg Gynecol Obstet 60: 55–64, 1935.
3. Best RR. Cholangiographic demonstration of the remaining common duct stone and its non-operative management. Surg Gynecol Obstet 66: 1040–1046, 1938.
4. Burgess CM, Honolulu TH. Solution of gallstones. JAMA 114: 2372–2373 1940.
5. Behrend A, Steppacher LE. The hazard of retained common duct stones. Amer J Surg 87: 520–522. 1954.
6. Strickler JH, Adkins RL, Rice CO. Ether flush treatment of retained post-operative common duct stones. Minnesota Med 37: 490–497, 1954.
7. Alfthan O, Kohler R. Ether treatment of retained post-operative biliary tree stones. Acta Chir Scand 116: 437–449, 1958/59.
8. Admirand WH, Small DM. The physico-chemical basis of cholesterol gallstone formation in man. J Clin Invest 47: 1043–1052, 1968.
9. Way LW, Admirand WH, Dunphy JE. Management of choledocholithiasis. Ann Surg 176: 347–359, 1972.
10. Bills PM, Lewis D. A structural study of gallstones. Gut 16: 630–637, 1975.

11. Trotman BW, Ostrow JD, Soloway RD. Pigment vs. cholesterol cholelithiasis: comparison of stone and bile composition. Amer J Dig Dis 19: 585–590, 1974.
12. Trotman BW, Soloway RD. Pigment vs. cholesterol cholelithiasis: clinical and epidemiological aspects. Amer J Dig Dis 20: 735–740, 1975.
13. Takasawa Y, Suzuki N, Takahashi W et al. A study on the dissolution and disintegration of calcium bilirubinate stones, with special reference to effects of litholytic agents in human bile and to irrigation of bile duct in dogs. Tohoku J Exp Med 138: 383–395, 1982.
14. Leuschner U, Wurbs D, Baumgartel H et al. Alternating treatment of common bile duct stones with a modified glyceryl-1-mono-octanoate preparation and a bile acid – EDTA solution by nasobiliary tube. Scand J Gastroenterol 16: 497–503, 1981.
15. Sutor DJ, Wooley SE. The nature and incidence of gallstones containing calcium. Gut 14: 215–220, 1973.
16. Pribram BOC. Ether treatment of gallstones impacted in the common bile duct. Lancet i: 1311–1313, 1939.
17. Best RR, Rasmussen JA, Wilson CE. Management of remaining common duct stones by various solvents and biliary flush regimen. Arch Surg 67: 839–853, 1953.
18. Pribram BOC. The method for dissolution of common duct stones remaining after operation. Surgery 22: 806–818, 1947.
19. Best RR, Rasmussen JA, Wilson CE. An evaluation of solutions for fragmentation and dissolution of gallstones and their effect on liver and ductal tissue. Ann Surg 138: 570–581, 1953.
20. Editorial. Rev Surg 22: 405–406, 1965.
21. Andrews E, Dostal LE, Goff M et al. The mechanism of cholesterol gallstone formation. Ann Surg 99: 615–621, 1932.
22. Rewbridge AG. The disappearance of gallstone shadows following the prolonged administration of bile salts. Surgery 1: 395–400, 1937.
23. Danziger RG, Hofmann AF, Schoenfield LJ et al. Dissolution of cholesterol gallstones by chenodeoxycholic acid. New Eng J Med 286: 1–8, 1972.
24. Tao JC, Cussler EL, Evans DF. Accelerating gallstone dissolution. Proc Nat Acid Sci USA 71: 3917–3921, 1974.
25. Higuchi WI, Sjuib F, Mufson D et al. Dissolution kinetics of gallstones: physical model approach. J Pharm Sci 62: 942–945, 1973.
26. Higuchi WI, Prakongpan S, Surpuriya V et al. Mechanisms of dissolution of cholesterol gallstones. J Pharm Sci 62: 945–948, 1973.
27. Earnest DE, Admirand WH. The effects of individual bile salts in cholesterol solubilization and gallstone dissolution. Gastroenterology 60: 772, 1971.
28. Way LW. In vitro dissolution of cholesterol gallstones. Surg Forum 24: 412, 1973.
29. Motson RW, Way LW, Wong A. The effect of solvent flow and solvent concentration on gallstone dissolution in vitro. J Surg Res 22: 287–293, 1976.
30. Higuchi WI, Prakongpan S, Surpuriya V et al. Cholesterol dissolution rate in micellar bile acid solutions: retarding effect of lecithin. Science 178: 633–634, 1972.
31. Tamesue N, Tsuyoshi I, Juniper K Jr. Solubility of cholesterol in bile salt-lecithin model systems. Amer J Dig Dis 18: 670–678, 1973.
32. Molokhia A, Feld K, Tochinda M et al. Dissolution of model gallstones in vitro: implications for t-tube infusion of retained common duct stones. Gastroenterology 69: 849, 1975.

33. Lahana DA, Bonorris CG, Schoenfield LJ. Gallstone dissolution in vitro by bile acids, heparin and quaternary amines. Surg Gynecol Obstet 138: 683–685, 1974.

34. Lansford C, Mehta S, Kern F Jr. The treatment of retained stones in the common bile duct with sodium cholate infusion. Gut 15: 48–51, 1974.

35. Mok HYI, Bell GD, Whitney B et al. Stones in the common bile duct: non-operative management. Proc Roy Soc Med 67: 658–660, 1974.

36. Toouli J, Jablonski P, Watts J McK. Dissolution of stones in the common bile duct with bile salt solutions. Aust NZ J Surg 44: 336–340, 1974.

37. Britton DC, Gill BS, Taylor RMR et al. The removal of retained gallstones from the common bile duct: experience with sodium cholate infusion and the Burhenne catheter. Brit J Surg 62: 520–523, 1975.

38. La Russo NF, Thistle JL, Hofmann AF. Treatment of common bile duct stones by intraductal infusion of cholate: a controlled trial. Gastroenterology 68: 932, 1975.

39. Way LW, Motson RW. Dissolution of retained common duct stones. Advances in Surgery WP Longmire Jr (Ed), Chicago, Year Book Medical, pp. 99–119, 1976.

40. Wheeler MH. Dissolution of retained choledochal calculi. Ann Roy Coll Surg Eng 59: 153–157, 1977.

41. Christiansen LA, Nielsen OV, Efsen F. Non-operative treatment of retained bile duct calculi in patients with an indwelling t-tube. Brit J Surg 65: 581–584, 1978.

42. James OFW. Symposium on retained common duct stones. Middlesex Hospital, London, 1979.

43. Sohrabi A, Max MH, Hershey CD. Cholate sodium infusion for retained common bile duct stones. Arch Surg 114: 1169–1172, 1979.

44. Motson RW. Dissolution of common bile duct stones. Brit J Surg 68: 203–208, 1981.

45. Sonnenshein M, Siegel JH, Rosenthal WS et al. Recurrent choledocholithiasis following cholecystectomy, sphincterotomy and choledochoduodenostomy: successful treatment with chenodeoxycholic acid. Amer J Med 69: 163–165, 1980.

46. Sue SO, Taub M, Pearlman BJ et al. Treatment of choledocholithiasis with oral chenodeoxycholic acid. Surgery 90: 32–34, 1981.

47. Salvioli G, Salati R, Lugli R et al. Medical treatment of biliary duct stones: effect of ursodeoxycholic acid administration. Gut 24: 609–614, 1983.

48. Dowling RH. Management of stones in the biliary tree. Gut 24: 599–608, 1983.

49. Ostrowitz A, Gardner B. Studies of bile as a suspending medium and its relationship to gallstone formation. Surgery 68: 329–333, 1970.

50. Gardner B. Experiences with the use of intracholedochal heparinised saline for the treatment of retained common duct stones. Ann Surg 177: 240–244, 1973.

51. Gardner B, Dennis CR, Patti J. Current status of heparin dissolution of gallstones. Amer J Surg 130: 273–295, 1975.

52. Chary S. Dissolution of retained bile duct stones using heparin. Brit J Surg 64: 347–351, 1977.

53. Toouli J, Jablonski P, Watts J McK. Dissolution of human gallstones: the efficacy of bile salt, bile salt plus lecithin and heparin solutions. J Surg Res 19: 47–53, 1975.

54. Sim AJW, Campbell EHG, MacKay C. The effect of sodium cholate and heparin on gallstone dissolution in vitro. Brit J Surg 63: 154, 1976.

55. Hardie IR, Green MK, Burnett W et al. In vitro studies of gallstone dissolution using bile salt solutions and heparinized saline. Brit J Surg 64: 572–576, 1977.
56. Romero R, Butterfield WC. Heparin and gallstones. Amer J Surg 127: 687–688, 1974.
57. Garcia-Romero E, Lopez-Cantarero M, Arcelus IM. Dissolution of human gallstone with clofibrate. J Surg Res 24: 62–64, 1978.
58. Garcia-Romero E, Lopez-Cantarero M, Quesada A et al. The non-operative removal of retained common duct stones after biliary surgery with clofibrate. J Surg Res 26: 129–133, 1979.
59. Thistle JL, Carlson GL, Hofmann AF et al. Medium chain glycerides rapidly dissolve cholesterol gallstones in vitro. Gastroenterology 72: 1141, 1977.
60. Uribe M, Uscanga L, Sanjurjo JL et al. Medium chain glycerides for the dissolution of retained gallstone: success and side effects. Gastroenterology 78: 1281, 1980.
61. Gadacz TR. Efficacy of Capmul and the dissolution of biliary stones. J Surg Res 26: 378–380, 1979.
62. Mack EA, Saito C, Goldfarb S et al. A new agent for gallstone dissolution: experimental and clinical evaluation. Surg Forum 29: 438–439, 1978.
63. Thistle JL, Carlson GL, Hofmann AF et al. Mono-octanoin, a dissolution agent for retained cholesterol bile duct stones: physical properties and clinical application. Gastroenterology 78: 1016–1022, 1980.
64. Wurbs D, Phillip J, Classen M. Experiences with the long standing nasobiliary tube in biliary diseases. Endoscopy 12: 219–223, 1980.
65. Schenk J, Schmack B, Riemann JF et al. Treatment of choledocholithiasis using the transpapillary perfusion technique. Endoscopy 12: 224–227, 1980.
66. Jarrett LN, Bell GD, Balfour TW et al. Intraductal infusion of mono-octanoin: experience in 24 patients with retained common duct stones. Lancet i: 68–70, 1981.
67. Mack E, Patzer EM, Crummy AB et al. Retained biliary tract stones: non-surgical treatment with Capmul 8210, a new cholesterol dissolution agent. Arch Surg 116: 341–344, 1981.
68. Uribe M, Uscanga L, Farca S et al. Dissolution of cholesterol ductal stones in the biliary tree with medium-chain glycerides. Dig Dis Sci 26: 636–640, 1981.
69. Gadacz TR. The effect of mono-octanoin on retained common duct stones. Surgery 89: 527–531, 1981.
70. Cassat JD, Shannon GJ. Dissolution of retained common duct stones using mono-octanoin. A case report documented with cholangiography. S Dakota J Med 35: 7–10, 1982.
71. Venu RP, Geenen JE, Toouli J et al. Gallstone dissolution using mono-octanoin infusion through an endoscopically placed nasobiliary catheter. Am J Gastroenterol 77: 227–230, 1982.
72. Dawson J, Cockel R. Retained common bile duct stones: mono-octanoin or endoscopic sphincterotomy? Gut 23: 906, 1982.
73. Velasco N, Braghetto I, Csendes A. Treatment of retained common bile duct stones: a prospective controlled study comparing mono-octanoin and heparin. World J Surg 7: 266–270, 1983.
74. Minuk GY, Hodenagle JH, Jones EA. Systemic side effects from the intrabiliary infusion of mono-octanoin for the dissolution of gallstones. J Clin Gastroenterol 4: 133–135, 1982.
75. Cole WH, Harridge WH. Disappearance of "stone" shadows in post-operative cholangiograms. JAMA 164: 238–243, 1957.

76. Catt PB, Hogg DF, Clunie GJA et al. Retained biliary calculi: removal by a simple non-operative technique. Ann Surg 180: 247–251, 1974.
77. Mackie B, Frackowiak RSJ, Cembala JA. Residual bile duct calculi: dispersal by irrigation of common bile duct. Brit Med J 4: 737–738, 1975.
78. Castleden WM. Retained common bile duct calculi. Brit J Surg 63: 47–50, 1976.
79. Glenn WR, Hill WH. Common duct obstruction relieved by injection of a topical anaesthetic into t-tube. South Surg 14: 3–6, 1948.
80. Harris FI, Marcus SA. Common duct stone relieved by injection of nupercaine solution into t-tube. JAMA 131: 29–30, 1946.
81. Cotton PB. Non-operative removal of bile duct stones by duodenoscopic sphincterotomy. Brit J Surg 67: 1–5 1980.
82. Okuda K, Tanikawa K, Emura T et al. Nonsurgical percutaneous transhepatic cholangiography — diagnostic significance in medical problems of the liver. Amer J Dig Dis 19: 21–36, 1974.
83. Perez MR, Oleaga JA, Freiman DB et al. Removal of a distal common bile duct stone through percutaneous transhepatic catheterization. Arch Surg 114: 107–109, 1979.
84. Mack E, Crummy AG, Babayan YK. Percutaneous dissolution of retained common bile duct stones. Surgery 90: 584–587, 1981.
85. Bernhoft R, Pellegrini CA, Motson RW et al. Composition, morphology and clinical features of common duct stones. Amer J Surg 148: 77–85, 1984.

Percutaneous Extraction of Retained Gall-stones

Richard R. Mason

The technique of extraction of retained bile-duct stones was first described by Mondet,[1] in 1959, in Buenos Aires. It is interesting to note that the first description of operative cholangiography was also from Buenos Aires and was by Mirizzi,[2] who also gave his name to the syndrome of concomitant obstruction of the cystic duct and bile duct.

DIAGNOSIS

The diagnosis of retained stones is provisionally made by T-tube cholangiography between 7 and 10 days after exploration of the duct. This timing allows easier differentiation of stones from both air bubbles and blood clot, which are constant sources of concern in the interpretation of cholangiograms of all types. It is recognized that the use of contrast which is too dense can hide gall-stones (Fig. 6.1), and it is recommended that contrast density in the region of 100–150 mg I/ml is used in routine cholangiography, with further dilution if the duct is considerably dilated. A delay of a few seconds should be allowed between the injection and exposure of the film in order to allow any stones to come to rest. A moving stone may not be seen on the film. It is also important to obtain complete filling of the whole of the biliary tree, especially of the ducts within the left lobe of the liver. It may be necessary to turn the patient on to the left side and even to tilt the table head-down in order to fill the left hepatic ducts. Failure to obtain the "complete" cholangiogram illustrated in Fig. 6.2 will lead to intrahepatic filling defects escaping detection. The presence of flow of contrast into the duodenum is a vital criterion in cholangiography. Any obstruction or delay of passage of contrast into the duodenum may indicate the presence of a stone or other abnormality at the lower end and demands a detailed assessment.

RETAINED COMMON DUCT STONES   Copyright © 1985 by Grune & Stratton, Ltd.
ISBN 0–8089–1729–3   All rights of reproduction in any form reserved.

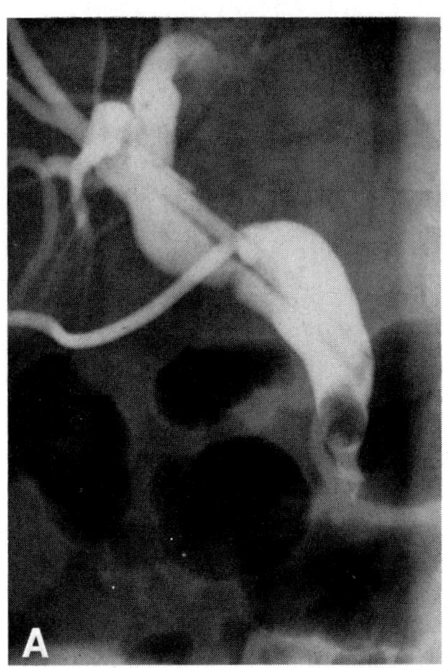
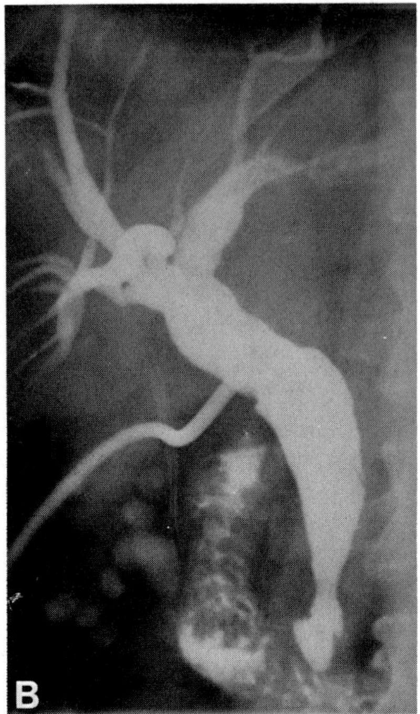

Fig. 6.1   The large residual stone seen at the lower end of the duct (A) is completely obscured (B) when the contrast density has been increased.

TIMING OF PERCUTANEOUS EXTRACTION

It takes about five weeks for a track to develop around the T-tube and for this reason manipulations involving the T-tube track are delayed, where possible, until five weeks after the operation. This interval can be safely shortened if the track is relatively straight and a large calibre (18 Fr. gauge or larger) T-tube has been inserted.

Traditional rubber T-tubes provide the requisite fibrous reaction for the formation of the track. Synthetic T-tubes are not advised.

PREPARATION FOR EXTRACTION

The reasons for the five-week delay have already been explained. Most patients can have their T-tubes spigotted and return home while waiting for their appointment for stone extraction. When the stone or stones are causing partial or total obstruction to drainage of the duct, a bile drainage bag must be provided. Many patients are able to manage such a system at home, but

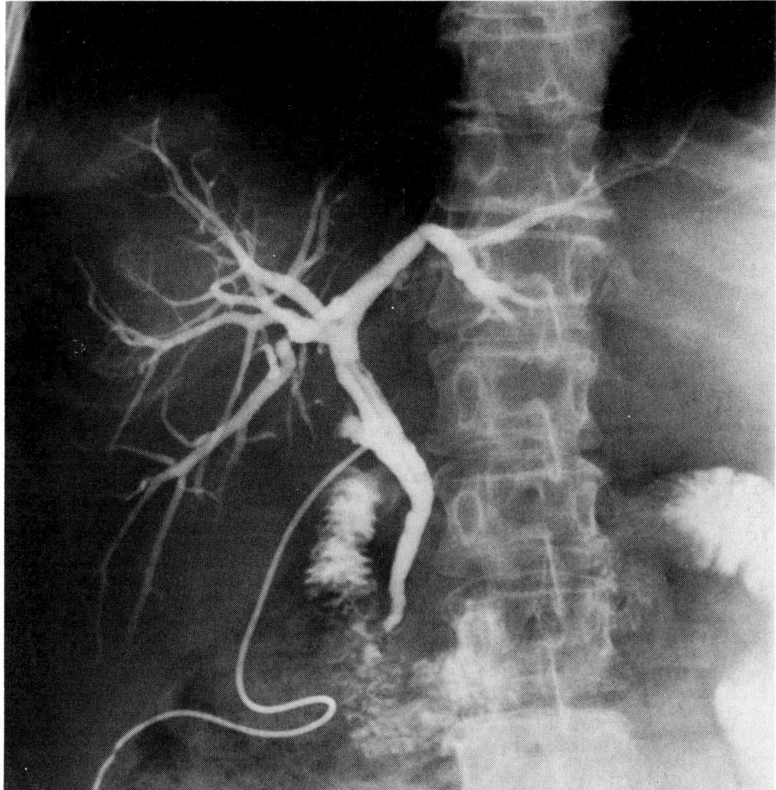

Fig. 6.2 "Complete" cholangiogram. It may be necessary to turn the patient on to the left side or to tilt the table head-down in order to achieve complete filling of the intrahepatic ducts.

older patients must often remain in hospital for supervision of their drainage system until extraction is performed.

Antibiotics

Antibiotics are only employed if the patient has had a recent episode of acute cholangitis, whether spontaneous or induced by T-tube cholangiography.

Explanation to patient

Only about half the cases can be managed by a single session in the x-ray department. If the track is difficult or there are multiple stones, more than one session may be required and this cannot always be predicted in advance.

As with all surgical techniques, time spent in explaining to the patient the details of the procedure, together with possible complications and, particularly, the possibility of multiple sessions, is well rewarded. Even if all the stones are removed at the first session, a straight tube is left in the duct (see below) for a completion cholangiogram on the following day. The patient should not be disappointed if an explanation is given of the reasons for leaving a tube after a successful extraction.

Anaesthesia

Most extractions are performed without anaesthetic of any kind. Patients are kept fasting for 4 hours before the procedure in case it becomes necessary to inject sedative and analgesic drugs intravenously. About 5% of patients need general anaesthesia (see below).

"Sterility"

The procedure must be regarded as a surgically clean rather than a sterile procedure. Nonetheless, the patient's skin is prepared and sterile drapes are employed as in a sterile surgical procedure.

Removal of the T-tube

If the T-tube track is relatively straight, the T-tube is removed just prior to preparation of the skin. If the track is slightly tortuous, or the T-tube is of small calibre (less than 16 Fr. gauge), the T-tube is cut short and left in position during preparation and draping. This allows the attempted use of a guide wire down the T-tube before extraction.

INSTRUMENTATION

Steerable catheter

Burhenne[3] has designed a steerable catheter (manufactured by Meditech) which contains four fine wires embedded within its walls. By pulling on the wires proximally, flexion of the tip of the catheter can be obtained in any desired direction. These catheters are available in 8, 10 and 13 Fr. gauge sizes and are suitable for most cases. They are expensive, but may be resterilized and re-used as long as they remain serviceable. They are not absolutely vital for the performance of the technique and any soft straight catheter (in combination with J-tipped guide wires where necessary) can usually be made to reach the stone.

Baskets

The baskets are of the traditional Dormia design and again the most commonly used are those manufactured by Meditech. These are available in three sizes and, like the original Dormia baskets for ureteric stone extraction, are introduced closed within their own sheath and are opened under x-ray control alongside the stone.

The disadvantages of these baskets are related to the small number of wires (four) and their elongated shape when opened. To circumvent these problems, William Cook (Europe) Ltd. has designed a prototype 10-wire basket which has a nearly spherical shape. This will ultimately be available in two sizes and is expected to facilitate extraction of stones from difficult locations.

EXTRACTION TECHNIQUE

In the original procedure described by Mondet[1] and continued by Mazzari- ello,[4] pliable forceps were used down the track for stone extraction. The ureteric stone basket was first used for this purpose by Lagrave.[5] Forceps are used very little outside South America and the stone extraction basket has received widespread acceptance. The technique is illustrated in Figs 6.3 and 6.4.

After preparation of the patient (as described above), and under x-ray screening control, the steerable catheter is introduced from the skin into the track of the T-tube. If the T-tube has been removed over a guide wire, the steerable catheter is, of course, introduced over that wire. Contrast is injected through the catheter to outline the entire track. The catheter is advanced under screening control until its tip lies just within the bile duct. The catheter tip is then deflected and the catheter advanced to a position alongside or just beyond the stone. Care is taken not to impact the stone, either in the region of the ampulla or in an intrahepatic duct.

A basket is then chosen according to the following criteria:

(1) Size. The basket size should be such that the maximum diameter of the basket is at least as great as the diameter of the duct. This ensures that when the basket is opened, the stone has no route of escape between the basket wires and the duct wall.

(2) Shape. The standard elongated basket is satisfactory in most in- stances. A spherical basket should be available for stones at the extreme lower end of the duct (to avoid unnecessary projection of the basket tip into the duodenum) and when the stone is close to the choledochotomy.

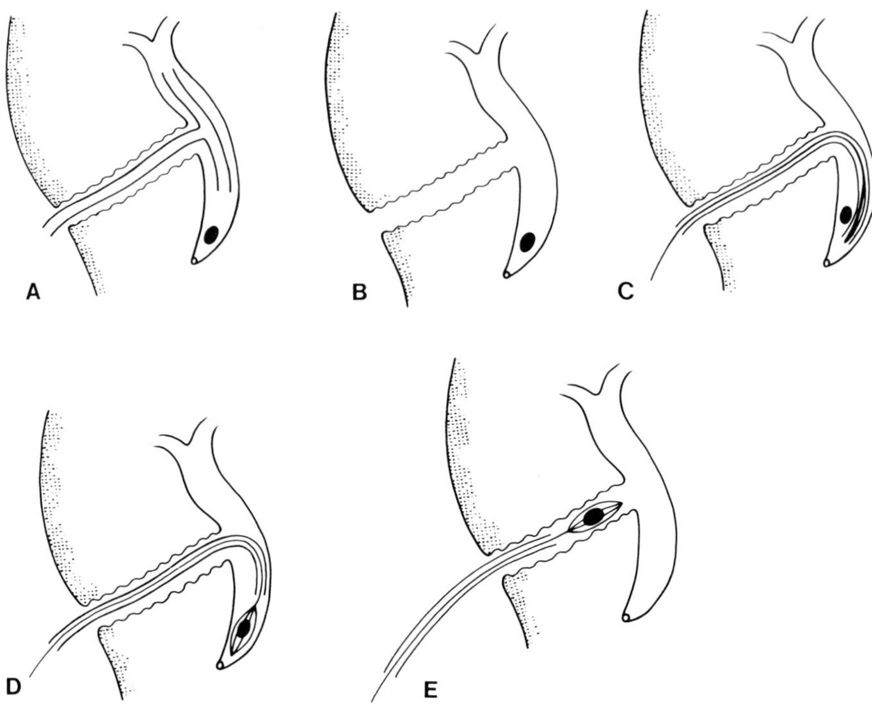

Fig. 6.3 Schematic representation of standard technique. (A) Post-operative situation showing T-tube and residual stone. (B) The T-tube has been removed, leaving a
track from skin to duct. (C) The steerable catheter has been introduced with its tip
positioned just below the stone, and the closed basket has been introduced through
this catheter. (D) The steerable catheter is withdrawn, allowing the basket to open
and the stone to be engaged. (E) The stone is extracted through the track.

The basket is now introduced, closed within its sheath, down the steerable
catheter and its tip allowed to project just out of the catheter. The basket's
sheath is then retracted allowing the basket partially to open within the
steerable catheter. Under precise screening control, the steerable catheter is
then withdrawn, and the basket tip (clearly visible because of the metal
marker) is not allowed to withdraw with the catheter. At this point, the
basket's wires spring open and short up and down excursions of the basket,
combined with rotary movements if necessary, engage the stone in the
basket. The basket is then withdrawn slowly into the catheter and as soon as
resistance is felt withdrawal is stopped. This manoeuvre enables the stone to
be grasped securely by the basket/catheter system but prevents shattering of
the stone which is highly undesirable.

The relationship of the basket, stone, and steerable catheter is kept constant

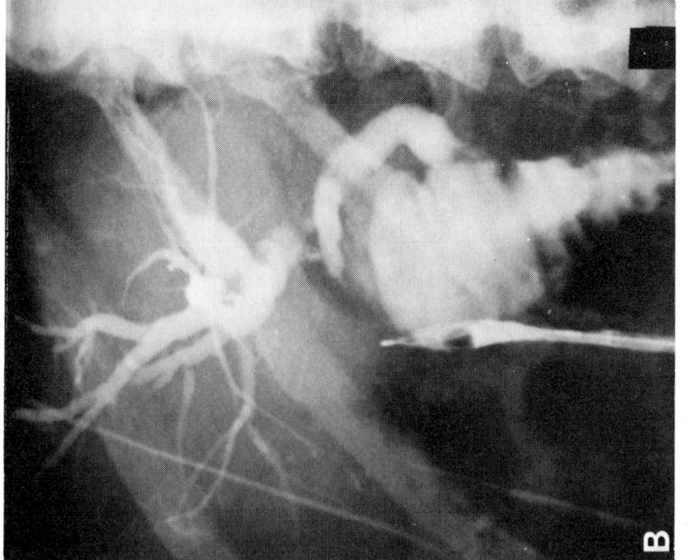

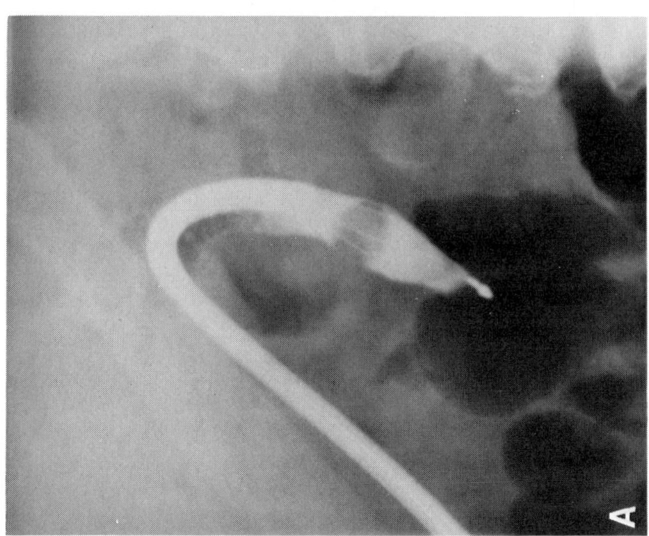

Fig. 6.4   X-rays taken during an extraction procedure. (A) The stone has been engaged in the basket within the common bile duct. (B) The stone is being extracted through the T-tube track.

by gripping the basket and catheter with one hand. The other hand then provides constant sustained traction on the steerable catheter at the skin, and the stone is delivered along the track on to the surface. If there are multiple stones, the procedure is repeated. Care is taken during subsequent insertions of the catheter along the track, as the prior extraction of stones may have caused some disruption of the lining. Again, contrast injection ahead of the catheter is vital for accurate steering to avoid the creation of a false track.

When all the stones have been removed (or the operator or patient wants to finish the procedure for that day), it is necessary to leave a straight catheter in the duct. Usually this catheter can be inserted directly. However, if the track is tortuous the steerable catheter is repositioned within the duct, a guide wire passed through it, the steerable catheter removed, and the straight catheter passed over the guide wire. We favour the use of endotracheal tube suction catheters for this purpose. They are available in 10, 12, 14 and 16 Fr. gauge, have an end hole and a distal side hole, and are just rigid enough for the purpose.

The catheter is spigotted overnight unless there are residual stones in the distal duct or extensive manipulation in the region of the ampulla has been performed. In these cases, the catheter is connected to a drainage bag.

If the catheter is spigotted, great care is taken to exclude air from the catheter before the spigot is inserted. We prefer the use of 3-way taps at the end of this catheter: saline or contrast is flushed through the catheter and the tap is then closed before the syringe is removed. The advantage of this technique is appreciated the following day when check cholangiography is performed. If air bubbles are left within the catheter, these are perforce introduced into the biliary tree during contrast examination, exposing the patient and the radiologist to misinterpretation of the filling defects so produced.

A very small dressing (5×5 cm) is placed around the catheter at its exit point from the track, a loop is made in the catheter around the dressing, and both dressing and catheter are secured to the skin with Opsite. This method usually results in secure retention of the catheter and a suture is seldom required. The patient, however, is warned to notify the nursing staff during the night if the catheter "feels different" as this may indicate that it is slipping out.

Check cholangiography

Check cholangiography is undertaken the day after the manipulation in order to allow air bubbles and blood clots, if any, to dissipate.

If the check cholangiogram shows no residual stones and there is free flow of contrast into the duodenum, the straight tube is removed in the x-ray department and a dry dressing placed over the opening in the skin. The patient can be discharged as soon as is convenient for him and he is given a supply of dry dressings and adhesive tape, with instructions to renew the dressing as it becomes damp and to notify his doctor if bile leak continues beyond 48 hours.

If the check cholangiogram reveals the presence of further stones or stone fragments, another extraction procedure is performed.

PROBLEMS

Problems relate to the track or the stone.

Track

The calibre and shape of the track are, of course, determined by the surgeon. Circumstances for percutaneous extraction of stones are most favourable when the T-tube is brought out straight to the right flank and is of a calibre at least as large as the stone (Fig. 6.5).

(a) *Tortuous track*   A tortuous track is more liable to be lost during manipulation, especially if multiple stones are present, and as a result multiple entries to the duct are required (Fig. 6.6).

(b) *Small-calibre track*   Small-calibre T-tubes contribute to the track/stone disparity problem discussed below. Furthermore, because small T-tubes are less stiff than large ones, small-calibre tracks (14 Fr. gauge or less) tend in themselves to be tortuous. They are much more likely to be lost during negotiation and false passages are easily created.

(c) *Anterior track*   Anterior tracks tend to join the bile duct at an acute angle. This angle is often difficult to negotiate with the steerable catheter. Furthermore, the radiologist cannot keep his fingers out of the primary x-ray beam as easily as he can when the track is a lateral one. For this reason, he is less likely to persist to a successful outcome when manipulation through an anterior track is difficult.

Stone

(a) *Size*   Large stones (i.e. larger than the track calibre) pose a particular problem (Fig. 6.7) because of the risk of fragmenting the stone. This converts a straightforward procedure of extraction of a solitary stone into a

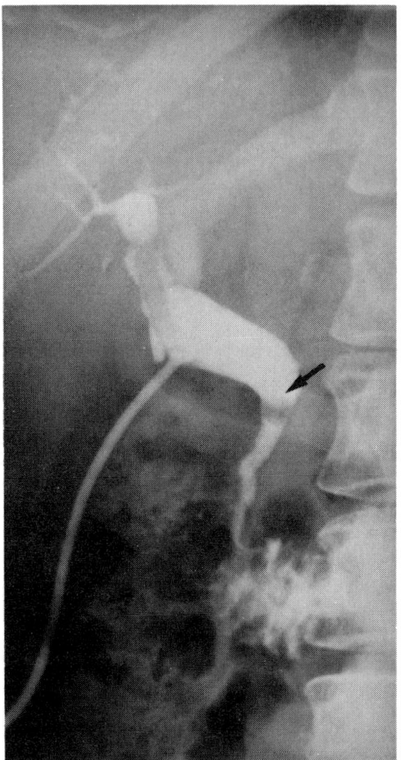

Fig. 6.5 The ideal case. The T-tube is at least 16 Fr. gauge and there is a solitary stone (arrow), no larger than the T-tube, in an accessible position.

near impossible situation of extraction of a number of small fragments. For this reason, when there is a considerable disparity between stone and track size, formal dilatation of the track is usually performed before extraction. This is likely to require general anaesthesia and the instrumentation for dilatation for percutaneous renal stone extraction has been found to be suitable. Dilatation can be performed safely up to about 26 Fr. gauge and, if there are multiple stones, an Amplatz sheath can be used (Fig. 6.8). After dilatation it is usually advisable to leave a large-calibre straight tube in the track (the same size as the largest dilator employed) for a few days to allow the track to heal at its new enlarged calibre. The stone can then be extracted according to the technique described without anaesthesia.

It must be recognized that there is a limit to the resolution of the film and television systems employed in the x-ray department. The resolution of the television system is inferior to that of film. Small stones visible on the films

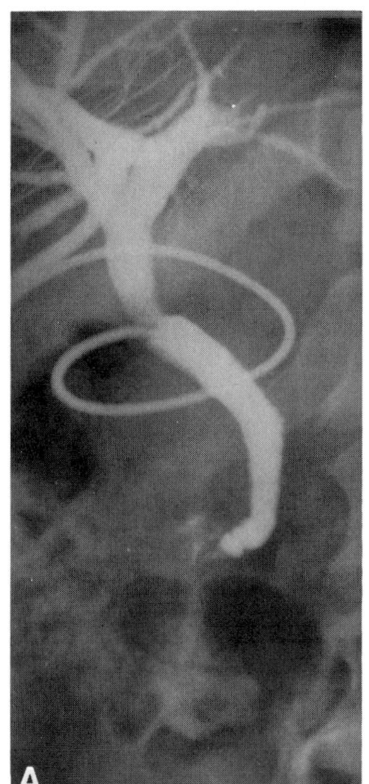
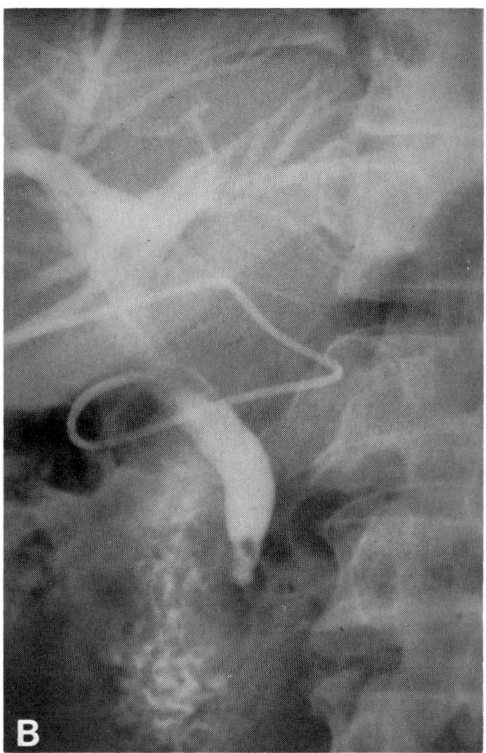

Fig. 6.6   Two examples of tortuous T-tubes tracks which make stone extraction difficult or impossible.

therefore may be quite undetectable on the television monitor. In any case, the resolution of the film system probably does not permit the reliable detection of stones or fragments less than 4 mm in size. When small stones or fragments are present and they cannot be engaged in the basket, we occasionally employ the technique of balloon dilatation of the sphincter to about 6 mm (Fig. 6.9).[6] This is followed immediately by rapid flushing with the catheter tip positioned about 2 cm above the sphincter. We have not used the suction catheter technique described by Magill and Baker.[7] Some

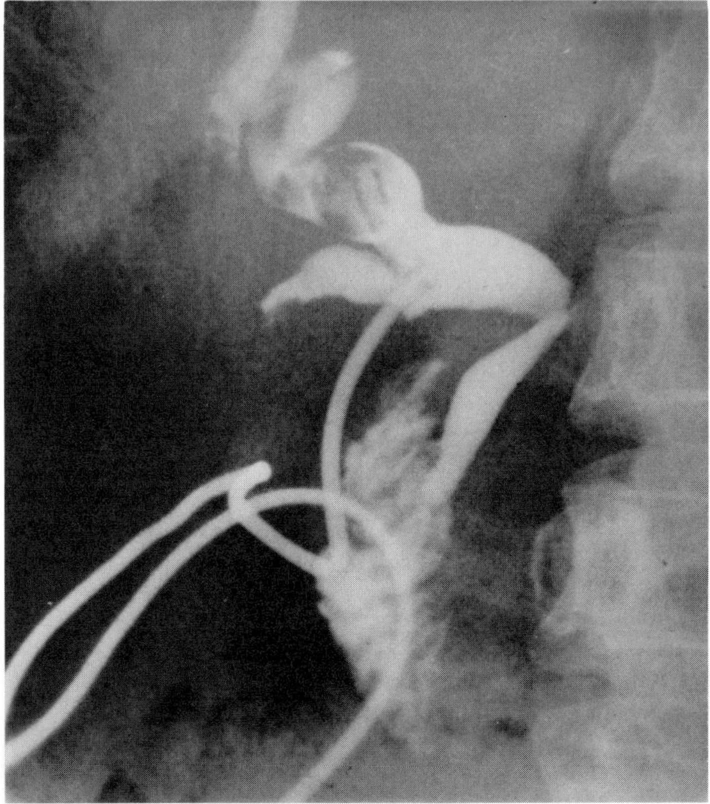

Fig. 6.7 A very large common hepatic duct stone unsuitable for percutaneous extraction.

patients are undoubtedly left with small stones or fragments after the T-tube track has closed. It is assumed that most of these pass spontaneously, but a possible relationship to late recurrent stones cannot be denied.

(b) *Location*   At least 80% of retained stones are situated in the extrahepatic bile duct. Most of the remaining intrahepatic stones can be dealt with easily as the stones really have nowhere to escape if the basket is positioned appropriately. Occasionally, small stones are situated peripherally in a non-dilated system and the problems associated with these may be formidable. The problems result chiefly because the catheter is required to be manipulated around sharp angles in a non-dilated system. Furthermore the television monitor image is, of course, two-dimensional although the biliary tree ramifies in three dimensions. Percutaneous transhepatic manoeuvres

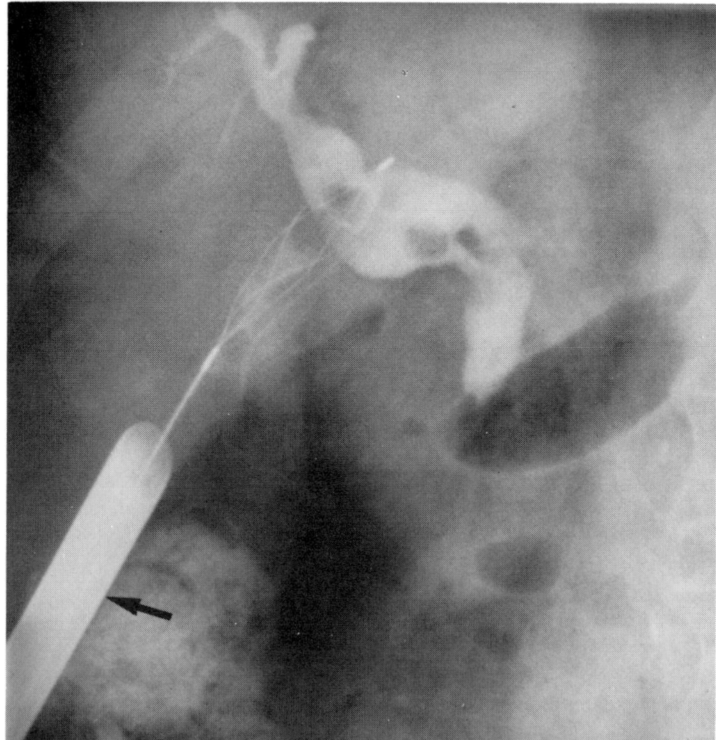

Fig. 6.8 Part of the track is supported by an Amplatz sheath (arrow). This reduces the likelihood of the track being lost when a number of stones require extraction as in this case.

should be considered if such stones cannot be extracted in the usual manner: if left, they are likely to produce complications in the longer term. A transhepatic catheter may push the stone into a more accessible position, or the stone may be crushed in a basket introduced by the transhepatic route.

Management of the rare cystic duct remnant stone has been described by Willson and Mason.[8]

RESULTS

The success rate of percutaneous extraction of gall-stones depends on the experience of the operator and the selection of suitable cases.

The success rates of Burhenne[3] and Mazzariello,[4] approaching 95%, contrast markedly with the 70% success rate in a collected series from twenty

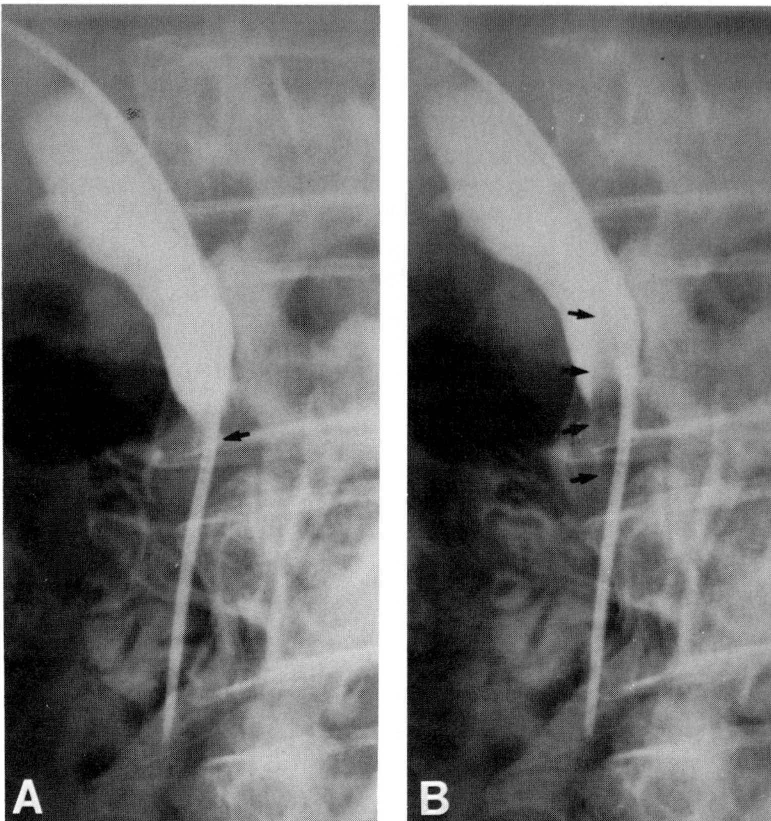

Fig. 6.9 Balloon dilatation of sphincter. (A) Balloon deflated (arrow). (B) Balloon inflated with air (arrows indicate the margin of the inflated balloon).

British centres.[9] Increasing experience of the operator clearly improves the success rate. Of our first 150 cases, 78% were totally cleared of stones by percutaneous extraction. Some stones or fragments were extracted from the remaining 22%, but endoscopic sphincterotomy was required in addition for complete clearance.

The ideal case is that of a solitary stone between 5 and 7 mm, situated in the common bile duct in a patient whose 18 Fr. gauge T-tube has been brought out direct to the right flank. Such stones can be removed within a few minutes without complications. Most patients do not, however, fit this description and success rates fall with multiple stones, small T-tubes, tortuous tracks and especially where tracks are brought out on to the anterior, rather than the lateral, abdominal wall.

The acceptance of cases which can be predicted to be difficult will understandably reduce the success rate. The availability of other non-operative techniques for retained gall-stones also influences management. We prefer endoscopic sphincterotomy as a primary measure in the following circumstances:

1. an urgent need for a result, when the patient will not tolerate the T-tube for the 3- to 4-week period beyond post-operative cholangiography, e.g. dementia, strong patient discontent;
2. when a stone is actually impacted in the lower end of the duct and the likelihood of successful percutaneous extraction is thought to be small (Fig. 6.10);
3. when the T-tube is very small and tortuous, especially if it is brought out anteriorly;
4. when there are small stones (less than 5 mm) in a dilated duct: these are usually very difficult to engage in the basket;
5. when the duct is very dilated, which is a relative indication for sphincterotomy, rather than percutaneous extraction, even if the stones could be easily extracted: this preference presupposes that endoscopic sphincterotomy can be regarded as a "drainage procedure".

COMPLICATIONS

Mortality

We are aware of two deaths directly attributable to this procedure, both resulting from acute pancreatitis following extensive manipulations at the lower end of the duct. There are at least 2000 reported cases of stone extraction in the literature and the mortality rate is therefore less than 0.1%. This contrasts particularly with the mortality rate of endoscopic sphincterotomy (about 1%),[10] and is the principal reason why we ask patients to wait a few weeks for percutaneous extraction rather than proceed to endoscopic sphincterotomy immediately.

Morbidity

(a) *Track perforation* Perforation of the track is a more likely complication when the track is tortuous and/or of small calibre. The track can usually be renegotiated after withdrawal of the catheter from the false passage and the stones then extracted uneventfully. Sometimes the track cannot be regained and injected contrast passes into the abdominal wall or occasionally into the peritoneal cavity. Loss of the track results in failure of the technique and is an indication for urgent management of known or potential biliary obstruction. We have employed endoscopic sphincterotomy with success in this circumstance. Emergency surgery or transhepatic biliary drainage may be required.

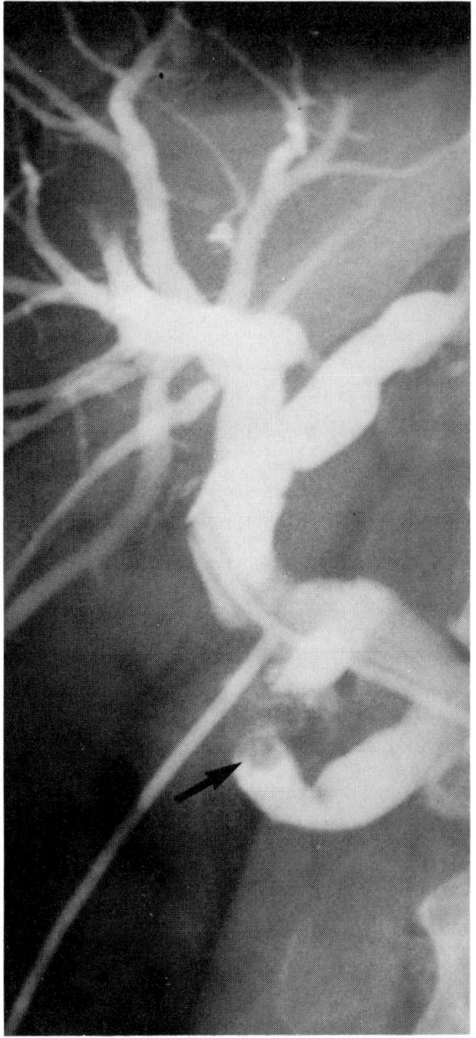

Fig. 6.10 A stone virtually impacted in the ampulla. The tortuous lower end of the bile duct prevents the basket from opening correctly and adds to the difficulty of extraction.

(b) *Fever* Acute cholangitis may follow the extraction procedure or attempted extraction, just as it may follow diagnostic cholangiography. Provided external drainage has been achieved by the passage of a straight catheter, the symptoms resolve quickly with antibiotics. The antibiotic cover should be continued for further manipulations.

(c) *Pancreatitis* Amylase levels have not been measured routinely following the procedure. Two patients in our own series (1.7%) had clinical episodes of acute pancreatitis, which resolved completely within a few days.

(d) *Stone lost in track* In our own series, two stones were delivered safely and successfully from the bile duct into the T-tube track but slipped out of the basket in the track between duct and skin (Fig. 6.11). These were known solitary stones in both cases. No further attempt was made to remove them and the patients remain well at one and three years follow-up.

Stones or fragments may also be removed from the track by re-engagement in the basket. This is essential if further stones remain in the duct.

The overall complication rate varies from 5 to 10% according to operator experience.[9,11]

OTHER MANIPULATIONS OF BILIARY DRAIN TRACKS

Gall bladder drains

The frequency of cholecystostomy as emergency treatment for empyema of the gall bladder is increasing, apparently with the increasing elderly population. At least 30% of these patients have bile duct stones demonstrated at subsequent cholecystostomy cholangiograms. The traditional management of cholecystectomy with duct exploration 6–10 weeks later, is now being supplanted by non-operative management of duct stones and any residual gall-bladder stones, without subsequent cholecystectomy.

Bile duct stones may be extracted through the gall bladder and cystic duct by a modification of the standard technique (Figs 6.12 and 6.13). The cystic duct may be difficult to catheterize but usually this can be accomplished with a combination of J-tipped guide wires and catheters with pre-shaped tapered distal ends. Usually the cystic duct also requires considerable mechanical dilatation before extraction of the stones, and for this purpose we use balloon-tipped catheters. Dilatation to 15 mm has been achieved safely at one session for extraction of large stones.

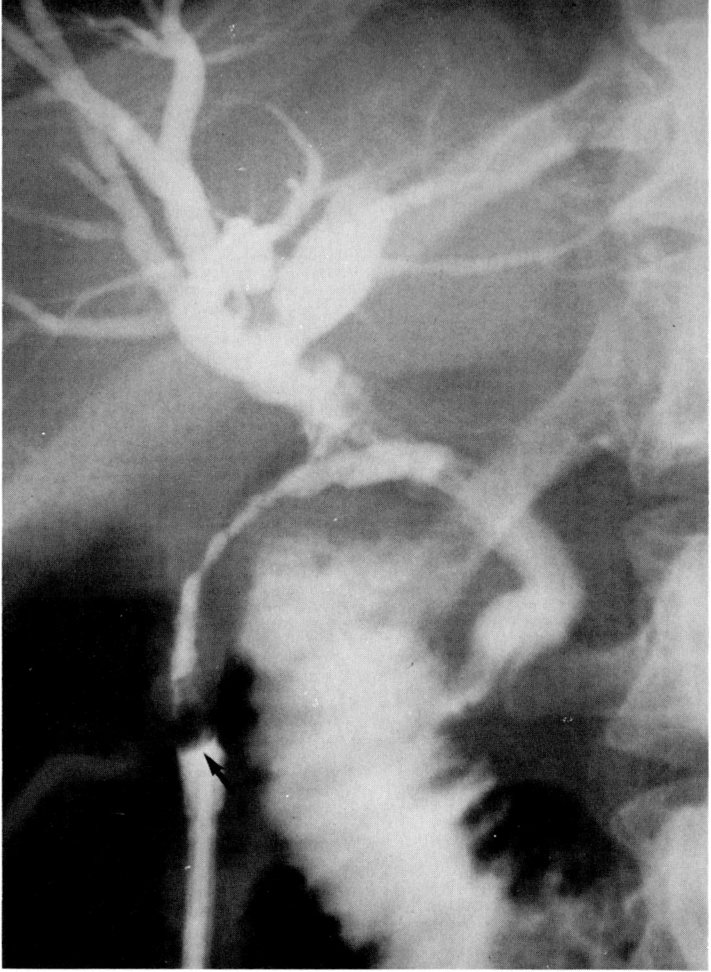

Fig. 6.11   A stone (arrow) has slipped out of the basket within the track.

Endoprosthesis insertion

The T-tube track provides a convenient and safe alternative to the transhepatic approach for insertion of stents (endoprostheses) through malignant tumours. Usually the upper limb of the T-tube is exchanged for a stent (Fig. 6.14). When the jaundice due to a malignant obstruction cannot be relieved at laparotomy, the surgeon should consider inserting a large calibre (at least 18 Fr. gauge) T-tube into the duct, either above or below the stricture, for subsequent stent insertion. The choledochotomy should be made as remote as possible from the tumour.

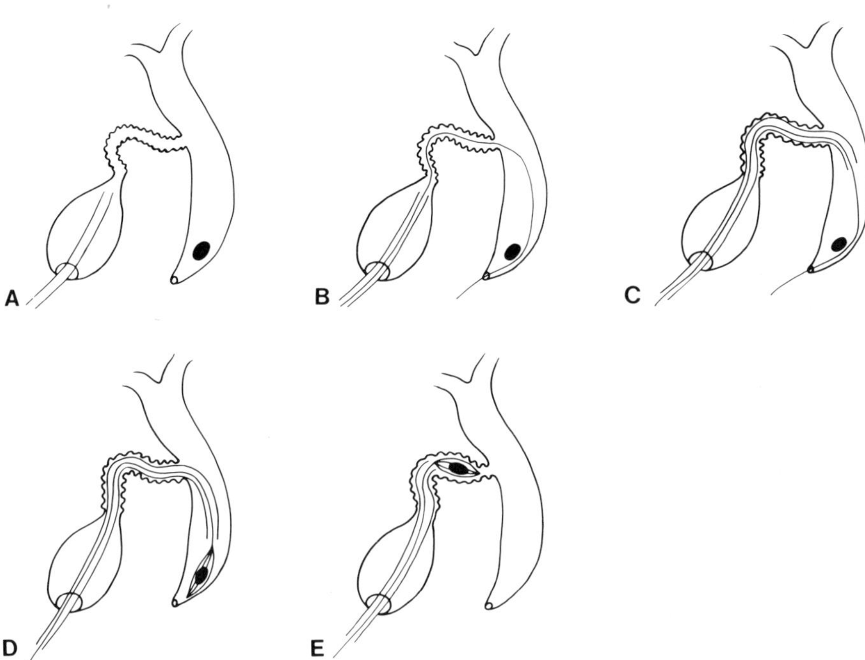

Fig. 6.12 Schematic representation of extraction of a bile duct stone via cholecystostomy drain. (A) The post-operative situation: cholecystostomy tube in place; stone in common bile duct. (B) The cystic duct has been cannulated through the cholecystostomy track and a guide wire passed through into the duodenum. (C) The cystic duct is dilated over the guide wire. (D) The basket is introduced and the stone engaged. (E) The stone is extracted via the cystic duct, gall bladder, and cholecystostomy track.

Catheter change

Our own success with residual stone flushing or dissolution is poor, probably because preselection of our patients has already excluded many who have responded to such treatment. We have occasionally employed T-tube track manipulations to position an infusion catheter directly against or above a retained stone (Fig. 6.15). A simple change of catheter may also be required occasionally for the purpose of obtaining an adequate post-operative cholangiogram of the intrahepatic ducts when this has not been achieved through the T-tube. Failure to obtain a "complete" T-tube cholangiogram is a particular problem after sphincterotomy, and when the lower limb of the T-tube has been left inadvertently projecting into the duodenum.

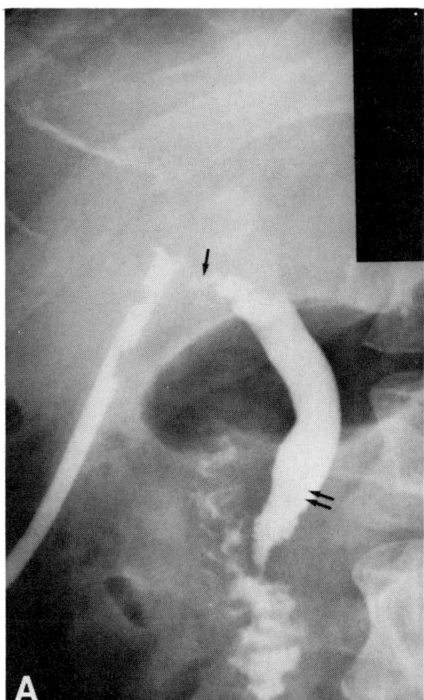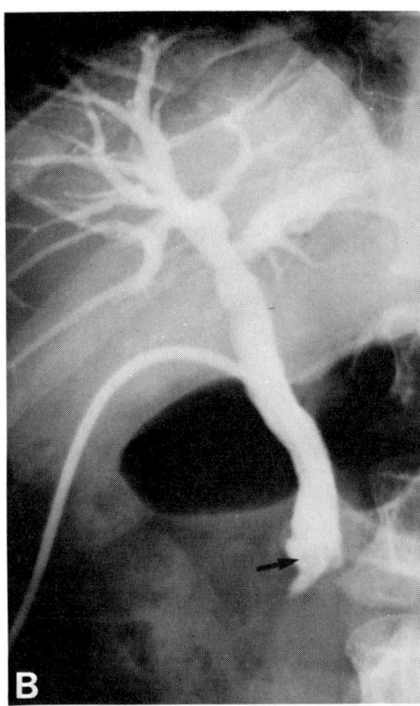

Fig. 6.13   X-rays taken during the extraction procedure via cystic duct, gall bladder, and cholecystostomy track. (A) Injection of contrast through the cholecystostomy tube outlines a very narrow cystic duct (arrow) and stone (double arrow) in the common bile duct. (B) The cystic duct has been cannulated and dilated. The steerable catheter is in position with its tip alongside the stone (arrow) preparatory to introduction of the basket.

In combination with endoscopic sphincterotomy

The variety of non-operative biliary procedures now available has allowed variations and combinations to be devised for individual patients with particularly unusual problems. These techniques include assistance for endoscopic sphincterotomy by means of wires or balloon catheters passed through the bile drainage track,[12] or through the liver,[13] and descending sphincterotomy.[14]

CONCLUSIONS

Although a quarter of a century has passed since the first description of extraction of retained stones through the T-tube track, the technique has

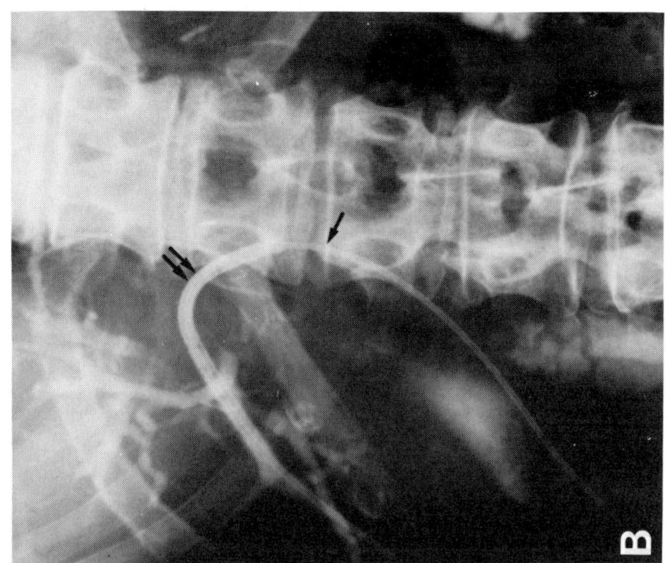

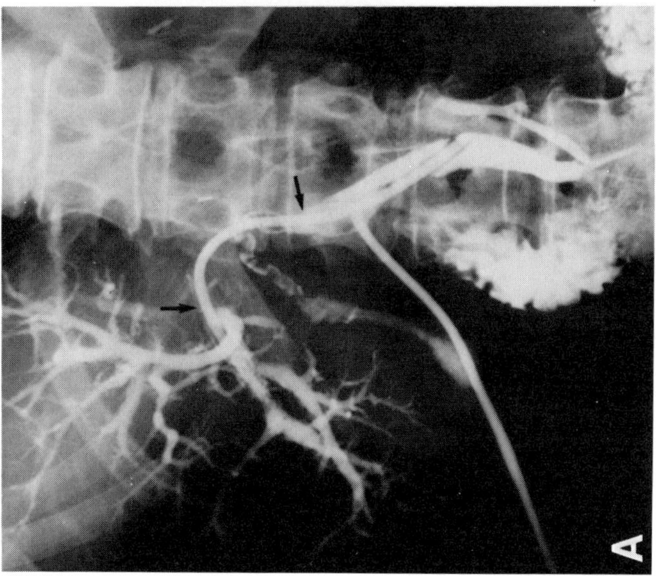

Fig. 6.14   Endoprosthesis insertion via T-tube track. (A) The upper limb of the T-tube has been passed through the tumour at laparotomy into the right lobe of the liver (extent of tumour delineated by arrows). Note complete occlusion of the left hepatic duct. (B) A standard 10-cm 12 Fr. gauge endoprosthesis has been inserted through the tumour. The guiding catheter (arrow) may now be withdrawn, leaving the endoprosthesis (double arrow) in place and allowing the fistula to close.

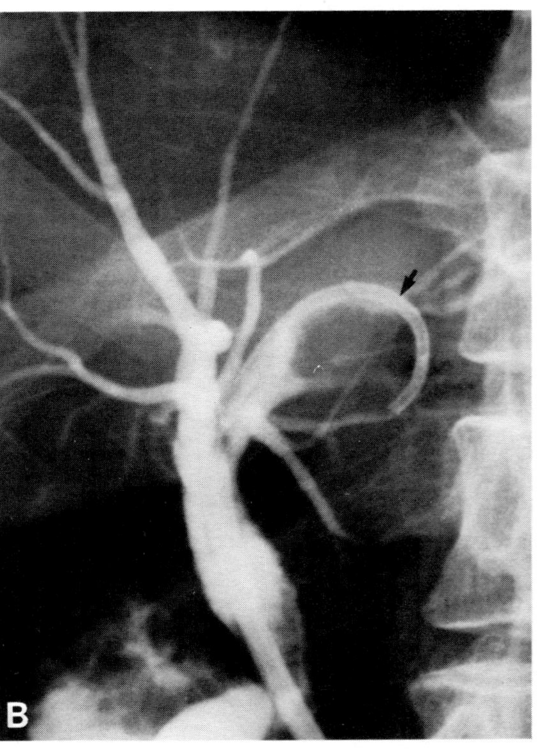

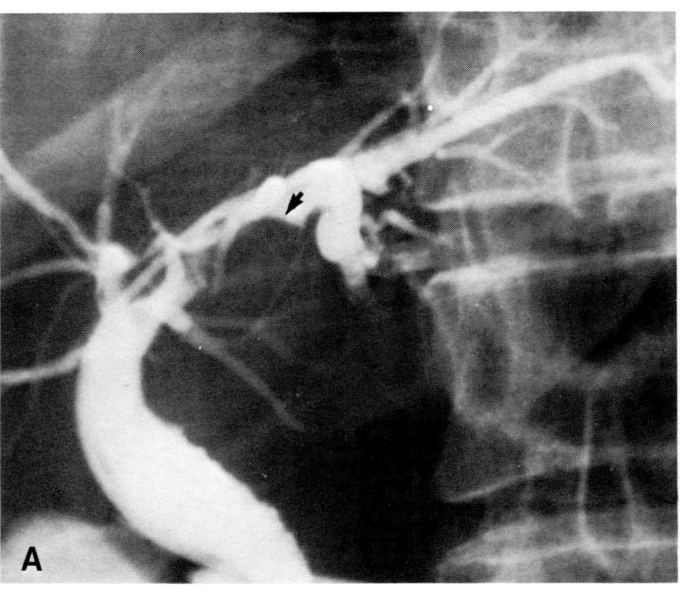

Fig. 6.15 Selective positioning of catheter for infusion of gall-stone solvent. (A) A large stone lies in the left hepatic duct (arrow). Basket extraction failed because of stone size. (B) A catheter with multiple side holes (arrow) in its curved distal end has been positioned around the stone for infusion of solvent directly on to the stone.

been widely available in the United Kingdom only for the last few years. It is unfortunate, in some ways, that its development in the UK has coincided with that of endoscopic sphincterotomy. Because sphincterotomy has the great advantage of immediacy, the relative mortality and morbidity rates have perhaps been given less consideration than they deserve when the individual patient with a retained stone is considered for treatment. Given ideal circumstances (and surgeons are very much themselves in control of these circumstances), T-tube track extraction is a very safe and quick procedure. Surgeons should be encouraged to use T-tubes of 16 Fr. gauge or greater, and in any case to use a tube which is at least as large as the largest stone which has been extracted from the duct. The tube should be brought out laterally, both to reduce the radiation exposure to the radiologist's hands and to increase the chance of successful extraction. Provided the radiologist is reasonably experienced, the success or failure of percutaneous stone extraction is largely determined by the actions of the surgeon five weeks previously.

REFERENCES

1. Mondet A. Tecnica de la extraccion incruenta de los calculos en la litiasis residual del coledoco. Bolletin Sociedad Cirujica, Buenos Aires 46: 278, 1962.
2. Mirizzi PL. Operative cholangiography. Surg Gynecol Obstet 65: 702–710, 1937.
3. Burhenne HJ. The technique of biliary duct stone extraction. Radiology 113: 567–572, 1974.
4. Mazzariello R. La extraccion instrumental de calculos biliares residuales. Boletines y Trabajas de la Sociedad Argentina de Cirujanos 27: 640–654, 1966.
5. Lagrave G, Plessis J-L, Pougeard-Dulimbert G et al. Lithiase biliare residuelle. Extraction a la sonde de Dormia par le drain de Kehr. Mem Acad Chir 95: 430–435, 1969.
6. Centola AP, Jander HP, Stauffer A et al. Balloon dilatation of the papilla of Vater to allow biliary stone passage. Amer J Roentgenol 136: 613–614, 1981.
7. Magill HL, Baker CRF Jr. A simple catheter suction technique for nonoperative retrieval of a retained common bile duct stone. Radiology 142: 788–789, 1982.
8. Willson SA, Mason RR. Inaccessible stone in the cystic duct remnant — a cause of failure of percutaneous extraction. Brit J Radiol 56: 492–494, 1983.
9. Mason R. Percutaneous extraction of retained gallstones via the T-tube track — British experience of 131 cases. Clin Radiol 31: 497–499, 1980.
10. Cotton PB. Endoscopic management of bile duct stones; (apples and oranges). Gut 25: 587–597, 1984.
11. Burhenne HJ. Complications of nonoperative extraction of retained common duct stones. Ann Surg 260–263, 1976.
12. Mason RR, Cotton PB. Combined endoscopic and percutaneous trans-cystic approach to a retained common duct stone. Brit J Radiol 53: 38–39, 1980.

13. Mason RR, Cotton PB. Combined duodenoscopic and transhepatic approach to stenosis of the papilla of Vater. Brit J Radiol 54: 678–679, 1981.
14. Mason RR, Shorvon PJ, Cotton PB. Percutaneous descending biliary sphincterotomy with a choledochoscope passed through the cystic duct after cholecystostomy. Brit J Radiol 55: 595–597, 1982.

7

Post-operative Choledochoscopy

Roger W. Motson

Extraction of gall-stones via the T-tube track, using a steerable catheter and stone basket under radiological control,[1,2] continues to enjoy a well-deserved popularity. The technique has been proven to be most efficient, removing over 90% of stones whether in the hands of radiologists who have done relatively few cases or in the hands of acknowledged experts.[3,4] Furthermore, the necessary equipment is not prohibitively expensive. Perhaps the only possible drawback is the radiation dose both to patient and radiologist, particularly when extraction is difficult and the procedure is prolonged. If the T-tube track is not in the preferred lateral position it may be difficult or impossible for the radiologist to keep his hands out of the exposed field.

The first reports of post-operative choledochoscopy came from Japan[5] and the United States[6] in 1975, and were followed by further encouraging reports during the next few years.[7-11] Introduction of the choledochoscope is similar to that of a steerable catheter, but once inserted the choledochoscope has the advantage that the operator works under direct vision.

TECHNIQUE

As with radiologically guided extraction using a steerable catheter, it is important to wait 4–6 weeks for the T-tube track to mature. Some stones may pass spontaneously during this time,[12] and the T-tube cholangiogram is therefore repeated to confirm that the stone is still present.

The choledochoscope is prepared in exactly the same way as for per-operative use, either by immersion in glutaraldehyde for 30 min or by sterilization with ethylene oxide gas for 24 hours. It is only the flexible choledochoscope that is suitable for post-operative choledochoscopy. Rigid choledoscopes are unsuitable, but an alternative which may be available in some hospitals without a flexible choledochoscope is the flexible fibre-optic bronchoscope. The outside diameters vary from 5–7 mm and it is therefore necessary in most patients to dilate the T-tube track before choledochoscopy

RETAINED COMMON DUCT STONES
ISBN 0–8089–1729–3

can be performed.[13] The dilatation of the track should be performed in the radiology department, with the aseptic precautions of skin preparation, sterile drapes, and sterile instruments. An angiographic guide wire is advanced through the T-tube until its tip lies in the common bile duct. The guide wire is maintained in position as the T-tube is withdrawn. A latex catheter, 2 Fr. gauge sizes larger than the T-tube, is then advanced over the guide wire until its tip is well within the common duct. The guide wire is removed and a check cholangiogram is taken. Dilatation is performed as an outpatient procedure at 3-day intervals; successively larger catheters are used until the T-tube track is sufficiently large to accept the choledochoscope (Fig. 7.1). On each occasion the angiographic guide wire is re-introduced before changing the catheter. This procedure should be performed under antibiotic cover.[13,14] A second or third generation cephalosporin is usually appropriate, but culture of the T-tube bile a few days beforehand allows accurate sensitivity testing and antibiotic selection.

The choledochoscope is introduced with the saline irrigation running to open up the T-tube track as the instrument is advanced. If any difficulty is encountered the guide wire can be re-introduced and the choledochoscope advanced over the guide wire, which then passes through the irrigation channel. Once the tip of the choledochoscope is within the common duct the guide wire is withdrawn. Alternatively, the choledochoscope may be passed alongside the guide wire.[13] Once within the common bile duct, the choledochoscope may be advanced both proximally and distally by deflecting the fully flexible tip, which angulates up to 120°, to lead the semiflexible part of the instrument into the common duct. When a retained stone is seen a stone basket is advanced through the instrument channel and passed beyond the stone, opened, and drawn back under direct vision. Once the stone is ensnared the basket is tightened to secure the stone (Fig. 7.2). The choledochoscope and stone basket are then withdrawn together. Stones high in the second and third generation of intrahepatic ducts, beyond the reach of the stone basket, may be drawn down into the larger ducts by balloon catheters.[7] If the stone basket cannot be advanced beyond the stone it may be possible to grasp the stone with tri- or quadropod forceps. Large stones can be fragmented either with forceps or the spiral stone basket, and the fragments then extracted or washed through into the duodenum.

On completion of the procedure an 10–20 Fr. gauge catheter, with two side holes close to the tip, is left in the common bile duct for 48 hours to drain the duct and allow further check cholangiograms to be taken. If many stones are present, or difficulties are encountered, the catheter maintains the tract open for further attempts at choledochoscopy. This is frequently necessary when there are multiple intrahepatic stones; sometimes many choledochoscopies are required before all the stones are removed. When

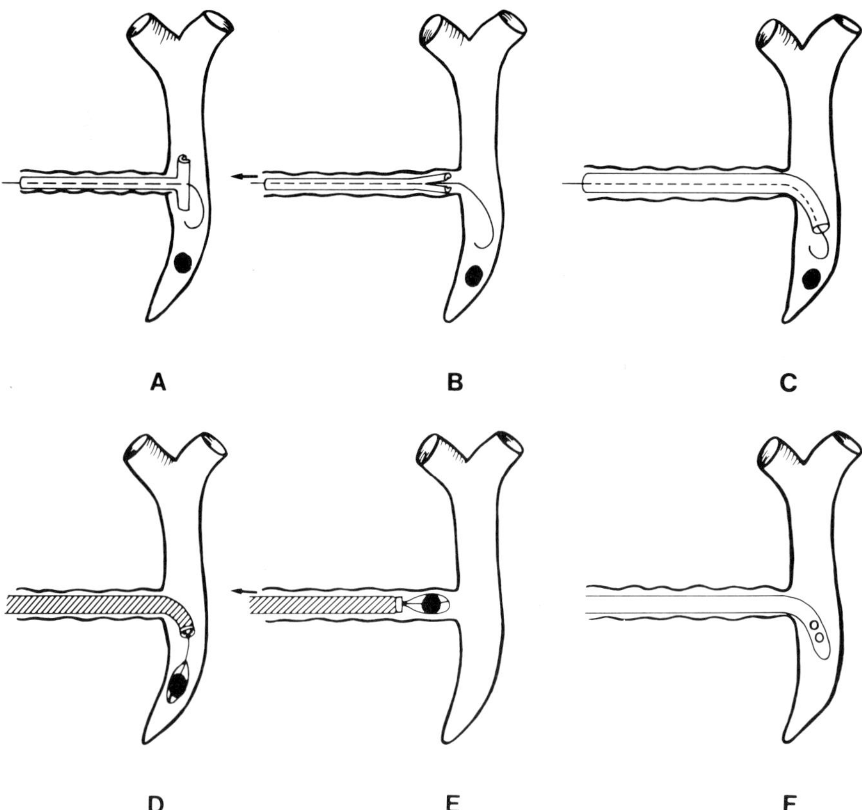

Fig. 7.1 Post-operative choledochoscopy. (A) An angiographic guide wire is inserted through the T-tube. (B) The T-tube is withdrawn over the guide wire and (C) successively larger catheters are introduced over the guide wire to dilate the T-tube track. (D) The choledochoscope is then introduced, and the stone visualized and ensnared in the stone basket under direct vision. (E) Choledochoscope, stone basket, and stone are removed together, and (F) an 18 Fr. gauge catheter is left with its tip in the common bile duct, maintaining the track open for drainage, check cholangiography or further choledochoscopy.

there is no doubt that the common duct is completely clear, the catheter is removed and the track allowed to close.

RESULTS

The results reported to date are encouraging and, although the numbers are not as great, the degree of success is at least as good as with radiological T-tube track extraction (Table 7.1).

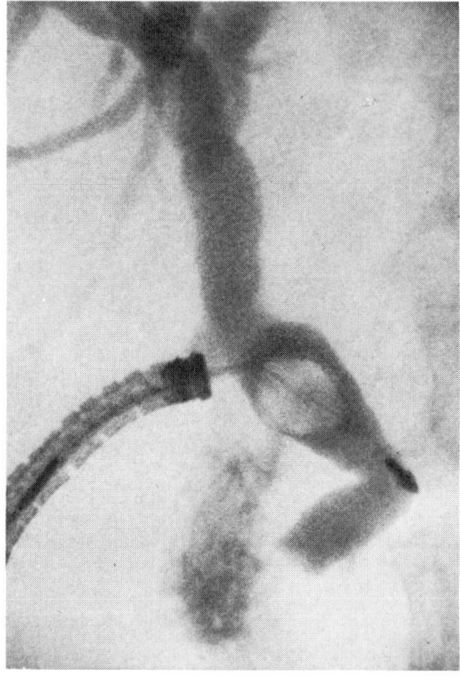

Fig. 7.2 Radiograph during post-operative choledochoscopy. The tip of the choled-ochoscope lies within the common bile duct which is filled with contrast. A stone in the distal common duct is ensnared by a Dormia stone removal basket. (Reproduced with permission from J. J. Jakimowicz.)

Overall, there has been complete clearance of the ducts in 311 out of 336 (93%) patients. In most cases the stones were removed at a single session. Some cases, most commonly those with intrahepatic stones, required multiple choledochoscopies to clear the ducts.[15,16] The slightly narrower and more flexible bronchoscope is probably the easiest instrument to use post-operatively, but the differences are not great.

Choledochoscopy probably has a slight advantage when the stones are very small. These can be difficult to see fluoroscopically, and when the steerable catheter is used a number of "blind" passes are sometimes necessary to ensnare these stones. Using the choledochoscope, the stone basket can be manipulated around small stones under direct vision.

Complications have been relatively infrequent. There is, as yet, no mortality reported. In Burkitt's series of 28 patients (not all with retained stones), pancreatitis occurred in two, vomiting in one, and pyrexia in seven.[14] Jakimowicz et al. had no cases of pancreatitis in 85 patients, though pyrexia occurred in 14.[18] Perforation of the sinus track occurred infre-

Table 7.1

Post-operative choledochoscopy for retained stones.

Authors	Year	No. cases	No. attempts	No. successful	Per cent successful
Sherman et al.[6]	1975	2	—	2	100
Gocho and Hirhesuka[9]	1977	4[a]	49	4	100
Yamakawa et al.[15]	1978	56	84	54	96
Yamakawa et al.[15]	1978	23[a]	367	20	87
Moss et al.[13]	1980	17	19	17	100
Hwang et al.[16]	1980	30[a]	129	25	83
Burkitt and Williams[14]	1981	22	26	21	95
Ker and Sheen[17]	1981	54[a]	425	49	91
Jakimowicz et al.[18]	1983	73	81	67	92
Berci et al.[19]	1983	55	>83	52	95
TOTAL		366		311	93

[a]All intrahepatic stones.

quently. Berci reports two cases in his series of 55, both of which resolved spontaneously, and Jakimowicz et al. had one case in their large series which subsequently required elective surgery to remove the stone.[18,19] A pyogenic liver abscess occurred in one of Hwang's cases of intrahepatic calculi — a patient who had previously undergone sphincterotomy.[16] Post-operative choledochoscopy has also been helpful in arriving at an accurate diagnosis in patients with stricture both benign and malignant, or polyps which resembled stones.

As with radiologically guided basket extraction, some patient selection is necessary. Very tortuous T-tube tracks may make it impossible to introduce the choledochoscope. The steerable catheter is more flexible than the choledochoscope, and negotiates very tortuous tracks more easily. One cannot expect very large stones to pass through a much narrower T-tube track. If this is attempted there is a risk of the stone slipping from the basket within the track, the choledochoscope and stone becoming stuck, or the T-tube track disrupting which may lead to a bile peritonitis.[20]

Dilatation of the T-tube tracks has not been difficult, but has been necessary in over 50% of cases in one series.[13,21] Use of large T-tubes should be routine. At least a 16 or preferably an 18 Fr. gauge T-tube should be used at the initial operation, no matter how certain one may be that the ducts are clear. It is only by assuming that every patient may require access to the common duct post-operatively that a T-tube of suitable size will be in place in the few who actually need it. A smoothly curved route to emerge laterally is ideal. If the common duct is not greatly enlarged then the intraductal portion of the T-tube can be trimmed down. In any case the backwall, if not already split, should be divided to allow easy insertion of a guide wire if this should be necessary subsequently.

The results accumulated so far are comparable to the early results with basket extraction under x-ray control. If the present rate of success is maintained as the technique spreads from experts to other interested choledochoscopists in the same way that radiological extraction has, then it will become an equally established technique for patients with the T-tube in situ. Avoidance of radiation to both patients and endoscopist, and being able to work under direct vision are considerable advantages, but dilatation of the track in a significant number of cases remains a disadvantage. In most series the patients have been admitted to hospital for the stone extraction procedure, whereas radiological extraction is often performed on an out-patient basis.

The two techniques should be regarded as complementary to one another rather than competitors. In many cases, neither will have a particular advantage, and choice will be influenced more by availability of instruments and expertise. In a relatively small number of cases one instrument may succeed where the other cannot. There will be very few cases indeed in which stones remain after employing both methods.

REFERENCES

1. Mazzariello R. Review of 220 cases of residual biliary tract calculi treated without reoperation: an eight-year study. Surgery 299–306, 1973.
2. Burhenne HJ. Nonoperative retained biliary tract stone extraction. A new roentgenologic technique. Am J Roentenol 177: 388–399, 1973.
3. Burhenne HJ. Complications of nonoperative extraction of retained common duct stones. Amer J Surg 131: 260–262, 1976.
4. Mason R. Percutaneous extraction of retained gallstones via the T-tube track — British experience of 131 cases. Clin Radiol 31: 497–499, 1980.
5. Mieno K, Noguchi T, Yamakawa T. Post-operative choledochoscopy and its clinical value. Jap J Gastroenterol 72: 1290–1297, 1975.
6. Sherman HI, Margeson RC, Davis RC Jr. Postoperative retained choledocholithiasis: percutaneous endoscopic extraction. Gastroenterology 68: 1024, 1975.
7. Yamakawa T, Mieno K, Nogucki T et al. An improved choledochofiberscope and non-surgical removal of retained biliary calculi under direct visual control Gastrointest Endosc 22: 160–164, 1976.
8. Moss JP, Whelan JG Jr, Powell RW et al. Postoperative choledochoscopy via the T-tube tract JAMA 236: 2781–2782, 1976.
9. Gocho K, Hirhesuka K. Post-operative choledochofiberscopic removal of intrahepatic stones. Jap J Surg 7: 18–27, 1977.
10. Okabe N, Kawai K, Kondo O et al. Operative and postoperative choledochofiberscopy Amer J Surg 137: 816–820, 1979.

11. Birkett DH, Williams LF. Choledochoscopic removal of retained stones via a T-tube tract. Amer J Surg 139: 531–534, 1980.

12. Bergdahl L, Holmlund DEW. Retained bile duct stones Acta Chir Scand 142: 145–149, 1976.

13. Moss JP, Whelan JG Jr, Dedman TC III et al. Postoperative choledochoscopy through the T-tube tract Surg Gynecol Obstet 151: 807–809, 1980.

14. Birkett DH, Williams LF Jr. Postoperative fiberoptic choledochoscopy. A useful surgical adjunct Ann Surg 194: 630–634, 1981.

15. Yamakawa T, Komaki F, Shikata J. Experience with routine postoperative choledochoscopy via the T-tube sinus tract World J Surg 2: 379–385, 1978.

16. Hwang MH, Yang JC, Lee SA. Choledochofiberoscopy in the postoperative management of intrahepatic stones. Amer J Surg 139: 860–864, 1980.

17. Ker CG, Sheen PC. Post-operative choledochofiberscopic removal of retained intrahepatic stones. J Formosan Med Assoc 80: 158–159, 1981.

18. Jakimowicz JJ, Mak B, Carol EJ et al. Postoperative choledochoscopy. A five-year experience. Arch Surg 118: 810–812, 1983.

19. Berci G, Hamlin A, Grundfest WS. Combined fluoroendoscopic removal of retained biliary stones. Arch Surg 118: 1395–1397, 1983.

20. Moss JP, Whelan JG Jr, Fry DE. Unsuccessful postoperative extraction of retained common duct stones: an analysis. Amer J Surg 135: 785–787, 1978.

21. Whelan JG Jr, Moss JP. Biliary tract exploration via T-tube tract: improved technique. Amer J Roentgenol 133: 837–842, 1979.

8

Endoscopic Sphincterotomy and Gall-stone Removal

Adrian R. W. Hatfield

With the development of endoscopic retrograde cholangiopancreatography (ERCP) in the early 1970s, it became possible to obtain precise radiological details of the pancreatic and biliary tree in a relatively non-invasive way. As many of the patients referred for ERCP had biliary symptoms or jaundice associated with common bile duct calculi, it was logical to apply the techniques of ERCP to develop a method for the removal of calculi from the common bile duct following endoscopic sphincterotomy. Initial results from various centres suggested the technique was effective and relatively safe, with a mortality of 1–3%,[1-4] but there was naturally some resistance from conventional surgical centres to accept this new endoscopic technique.

It is difficult to obtain a consensus of accurate current mortality rates for surgical exploration of the bile duct. This depends on the patient's age, general medical condition and previous surgery to the bile duct. In general terms, the mortality of bile duct exploration in patients under the age of 60 years is less than 1%.[5,6] However, in the elderly, with the medical problems that increasing age brings, the mortality rises progressively and ranges from 1 to 12%.[6-8] Multiple attempts at bile duct exploration are associated with increasing post-operative problems, and surgery in the presence of acute cholangitis increases the operative risk.[9] It is even more difficult to obtain accurate figures for the success of surgical removal of common bile duct calculi following previous biliary exploration, which is the situation for most patients undergoing endoscopic sphincterotomy. The retained stone rate after secondary bile duct exploration ranges from 3 to 33%.[8,10]

It is getting increasingly difficult to compare the results of surgery directly with those of endoscopic sphincterotomy, as patients undergoing endoscopic manoeuvres tend to be the elderly and medically unfit — the very patients who are turned down as representing too great a risk for surgery. However, the increasing demand for endoscopic sphincterotomy speaks for itself, and recent improvements to endoscopic equipment have produced better results.[11,12] and have lead to a greater acceptance of the technique.

It is now generally accepted that the elderly and medically unfit patient presenting with common bile duct calculi following cholecystectomy, should be managed by endoscopic sphincterotomy with gall-stone removal and not by a second operation.[13] The situations of younger patients and those with their gall bladders still in situ remain controversial, and are areas where the precise roles of surgery and endoscopic sphincterotomy are not yet clear.

INSTRUMENTS AND ACCESSORIES

A typical endoscope in use now is a side-viewing duodenoscope with an insulated tip, such as an Olympus JF-1T. The endoscope has an earthing terminal for patient and operator safety. The instrumentation/suction channel is large enough to take 7 and 8 Fr. gauge accessories. The degree of elevation of the bridge at the distal end of the instrumentation channel, and the flexibility of the four-way angling distal tip of the endoscope, allow for great manoeuvrability within the second part of the duodenum in the region of the papilla of Vater. Larger instruments such as the Olympus 3.7T can also be used, especially for difficult cases. Although they have a greater outside diameter, the 3.7 mm channel (10 Fr. gauge) allows 7 or 8 Fr. gauge accessories to be used and still leaves sufficient room for simultaneous aspiration of duodenal contents.

The most widely used sphincterotome is of a bow-string design (Fig. 8.1). This particular model has a single, stainless steel wire through which a cutting diathermy current is passed. As tension is applied to the wire via an instrument handle the catheter adopts a bow-string shape. Other diathermy catheters have softer, braided steel wires that can be easier to cannulate with, but which tend to burn through more quickly. A diathermy source that can administer both a cutting and coagulating current is necessary. Ideally, the diathermy unit should allow cutting and coagulation currents to be blended according to the individual patient's needs. The two types most commonly used are the Olympus PSD and the Erbe. At present, a bi-polar system is used incorporating a patient plate with a cut-out system if the plate is connected incorrectly.

There are many shapes and sizes of baskets for stone retrieval. Initially, versions of the Dormia type of basket, previously used in the ureter for retrieval of renal calculi, were used. However, most centres now use a "chinese lantern" type of stone basket (Fig. 8.2) which has soft, floppy braided wires which are less likely to trap and traumatize the bile duct mucosa than the spiral type.

Long, endoscopic balloon catheters have now been developed (Fig. 8.3) and these can be passed into and inflated within the bile duct. Those with

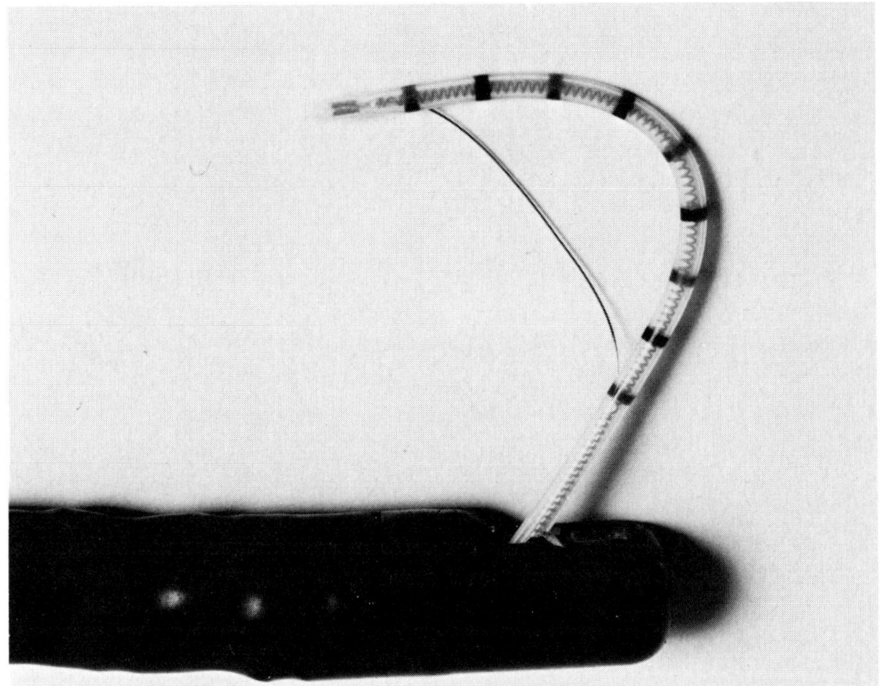

Fig. 8.1 An Olympus JF1-T duodenoscope. A bow-string type sphincterotome has been passed out of the instrument and the wire tightened into the cutting position.

softer, latex spherical balloons (Fogarty type) can be used for assessing the size of the sphincterotomy opening, and for removing small stones and gravel from the bile duct. Those with sausage-shaped balloons (Gruntzig type) are made of toughened vinyl and can be used to dilate up a fibrotic papilla or biliary stricture. Both these balloons are 7 Fr. gauge and can be passed over a 0.035 radiological guide-wire.

There is also a range of 7 and 8 Fr. gauge drainage tubes that can be left in the bile duct after sphincterotomy to provide drainage while large stones are passing.

TECHNIQUES

Patients are prepared as for conventional ERCP with an overnight fast and sedated with intravenous diazepan and pethidine if necessary. Patients should have an intravenous infusion set up prior to the procedure and ideally

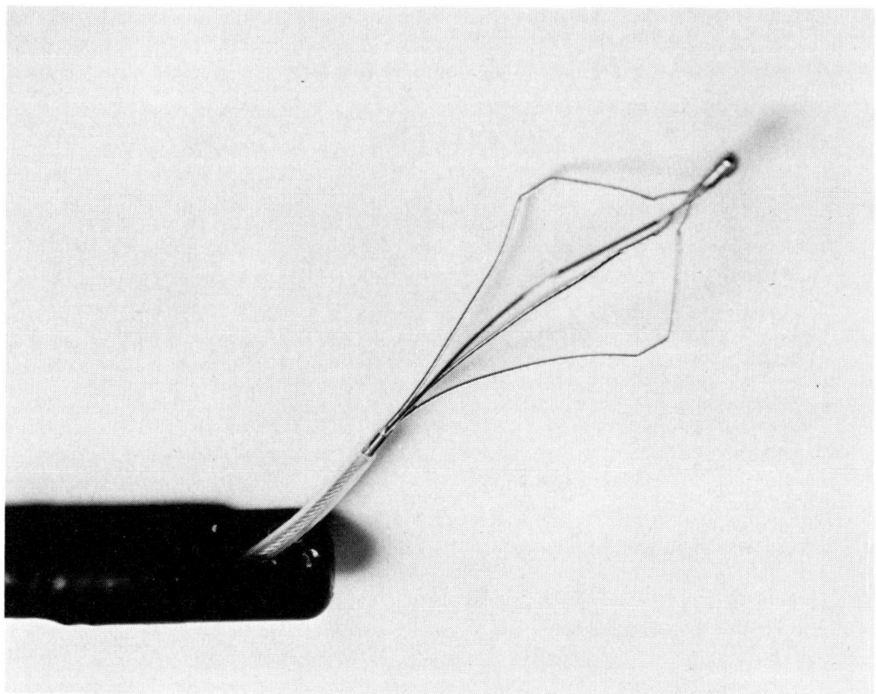

Fig. 8.2   An Olympus JF1-T duodenoscope with an open stone basket.

should have a normal haemoglobin concentration, platelet count and prothrombin index. It is unnecessary to routinely cross-match blood for the procedure.

Having opacified both the pancreatic and biliary duct systems and taken appropriate radiographs, the sphincterotome is inserted deep into the bile duct. On screening the wire of the catheter must be seen clearly to be in the bile duct and not in the pancreatic duct, or pancreatitis may result. A cut is made through the papilla in an upwards direction for about 1–1.5 cm until the inside of the bile duct is visible and the majority, or all, of the sphincter muscle has been divided. During this initial cut there may be a small amount of blood loss followed by a gush of bile. It is important not to cut too far otherwise severe bleeding or retroperitoneal perforation may occur.

Due to magnification of the endoscopic view, it is often difficult to judge distances accurately. Therefore to assess the size of the sphincterotomy orifice, it is advisable to insert a balloon catheter into the bile duct and pull the balloon, inflated to 1 cm, through the sphincterotomy orifice into the duodenum. Gall-stone extraction should not be attempted until an adequate sphincterotomy has been performed.

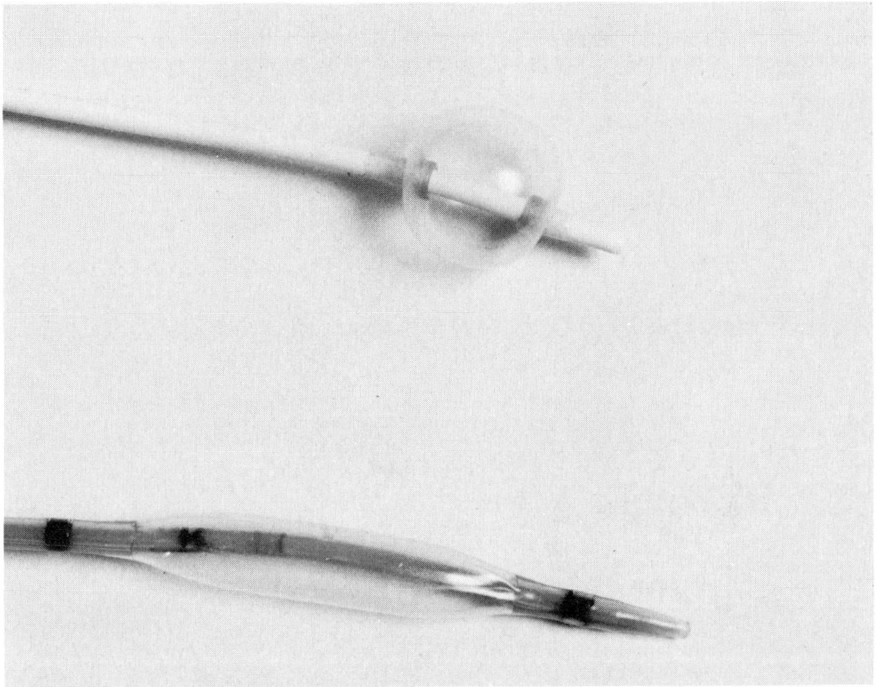

Fig. 8.3 Two types of endoscopic balloon catheter commonly used in the bile duct.
The upper catheter with a spherical balloon can be used for assessing the size of the
sphincterotomy and extracting small stones. The lower catheter can be passed over a
guide-wire and has a longer, toughened vinyl balloon and is used for dilating biliary
strictures and the papillary orifice.

Sometimes it is not possible to perform a full sphincterotomy on the first
occasion, due to difficult visualization, access, or papillary fibrosis. In this
situation a small cut is made in the surface of the papilla, a "pre-cut", and
the patient is then re-examined at a later date, at which time it is hoped the
duct can be successfully cannulated and a full sphincterotomy performed.

After performing the sphincterotomy, calculi can either be actively
removed or left to pass spontaneously. There is a tendency, especially in the
larger referral centres, to attempt to clear the bile duct of calculi at the first
procedure so that the patient can be discharged without the need for a
second procedure.

Small stones may pass spontaneously with the rush of bile after division of
the sphincter, otherwise they can be pulled out with minimal effort using a
balloon catheter (Fig. 8.4). Larger stones need to be trapped in a basket and
pulled out into the duodenum individually (Fig. 8.5). Following sphinctero-

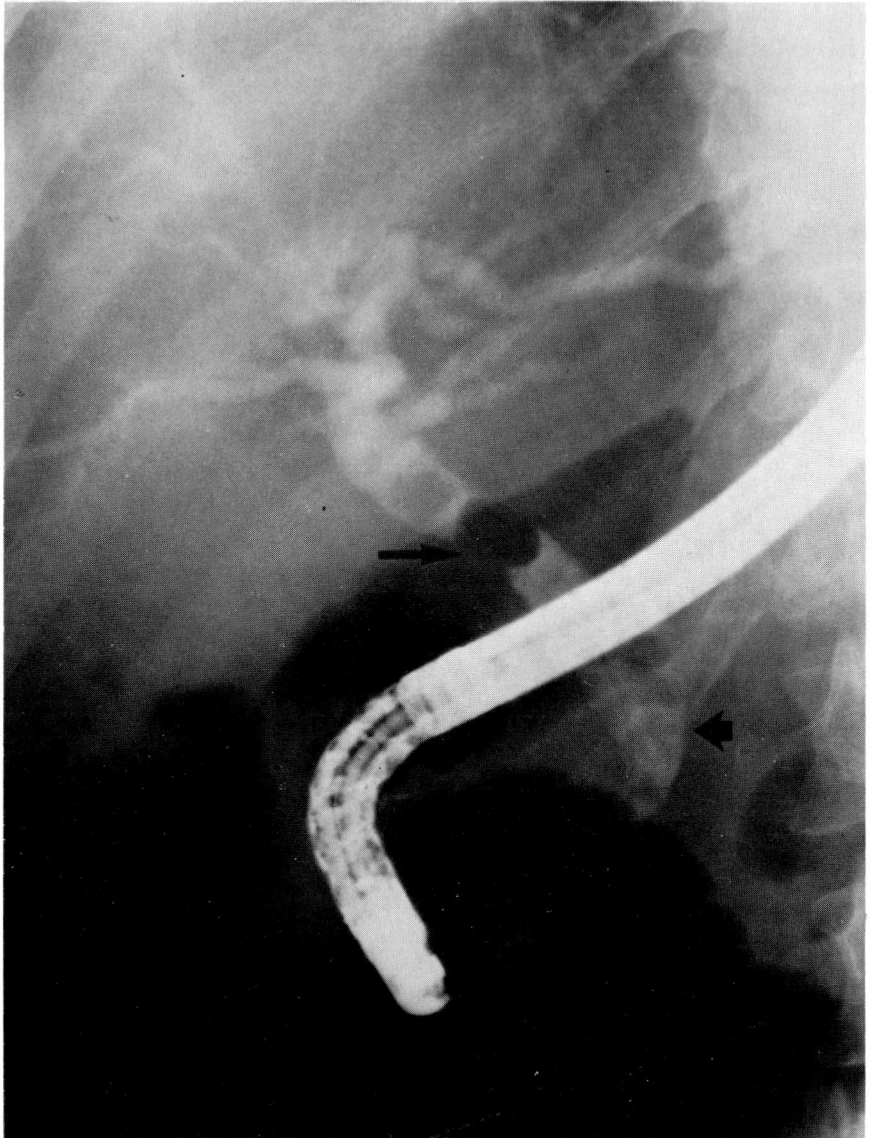

Fig. 8.4 An ERCP showing multiple small calculi in the bile duct (large arrow). A balloon catheter has been inflated (small arrow) above some of the stones, which can then be pulled out into the duodenum.

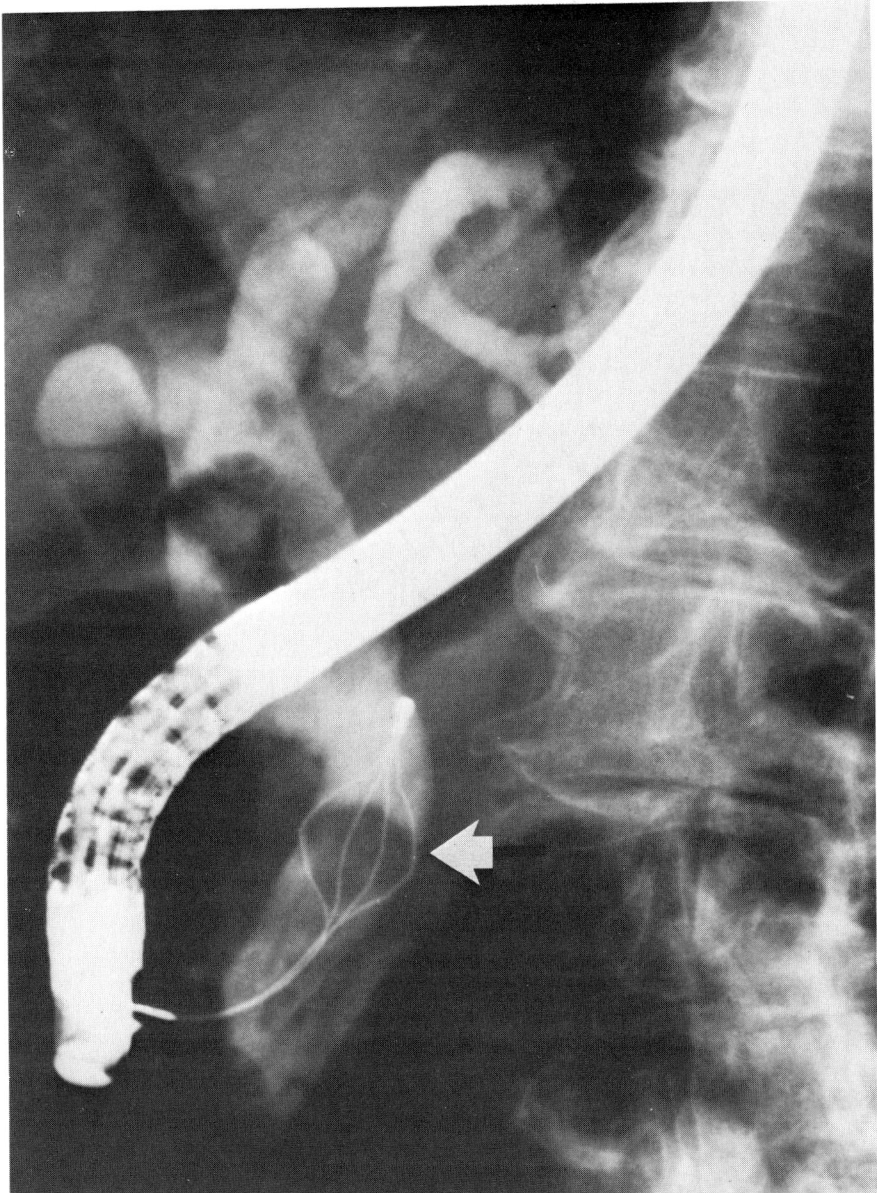

Fig. 8.5 An ERCP showing the lowest of several calculi in the bile duct, trapped in a stone basket (arrow) ready for extraction into the duodenum.

tomy and gall-stone extraction, the bile duct often empties of contrast and on x-ray is seen to be filled with air (Fig. 8.6). Solitary calculi are relatively easy to trap in the basket and remove, but care must be taken with multiple calculi not to trap a calculus high in the bile duct that might then impact and jam against a lower stone during attempted removal. With multiple calculi it is often advisable to wait for the subsequent spontaneous passage of calculi and, if necessary, re-admit the patient some weeks later for a further ERCP to remove any stones that may remain at that stage, enlarging the sphincter-otomy if necessary.

Calculi of up to 1–1.5 cm can usually be extracted quite easily from the bile duct with a basket. However, calculi of 2 cm or more, can present difficulties both in getting them into the stone basket and then removing them from the bile duct. On occasion, very large calculi of 2 cm do pass spontaneously once an adequate sphincterotomy has been performed. However, it is a mistake to attempt to extend a sphincterotomy beyond 2 cm in length as the chances of severe bleeding or retroduodenal perforation are extremely high. The problem of very large or multiple calculi that defy initial or subsequent removal will be dealt with later.

The policy for the use of antibiotics varies from centre to centre. In general, prophylactic antibiotics should be given, particularly if patients have had preceding cholangitis. After the procedure, antibiotics need only be given if the procedure has been complicated or the bile duct incompletely cleared of calculi. In our department, we would then use gentamicin or amoxycillin intravenously for 48 hours. The patient should also be kept to nil-by-mouth for 6–12 hours and the intravenous infusion continued for 12–24 hours. Most patients experience only minimal, if any, discomfort during the procedure and are usually ready for discharge within 48 hours, providing their course has been uncomplicated.

INDICATIONS

There seems little doubt that the major indications for endoscopic sphincter-otomy is gall-stone removal in the elderly and medically unfit patient with common bile duct calculi, either solitary or multiple, who has undergone previous biliary surgery either months or years before. Precisely what constitutes elderly or medically unfit will vary from patient to patient, but there is no doubt that the decision to choose an endoscopic route rather than surgery, should be mutually agreed between the surgeon and physician. At present, it is felt that as biliary surgery in the younger age group is associated with an extremely low mortality, endoscopic sphincterotomy should prob-ably be restricted to the middle-aged or elderly patients. In general, it is

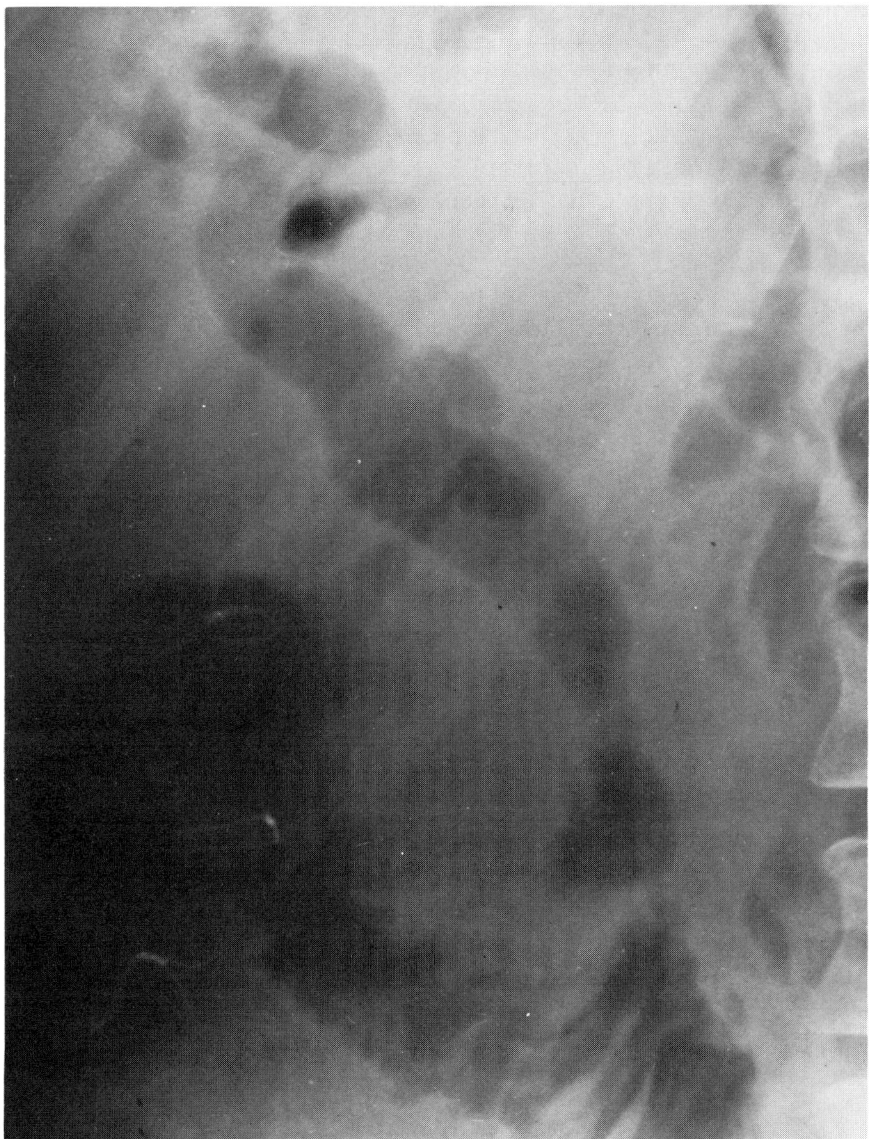

Fig. 8.6 A totally air-filled bile duct after endoscopic sphincterotomy and gall-stone removal.

possible to predict that complications after surgery will be more common in the older age group, whereas complications after endoscopic sphincterotomy, although few, can occur at any age.

When retained gall-stones are discovered on a T-tube cholangiogram following bile duct exploration, they can be extracted down the T-tube track using a steerable catheter, as described by Burhenne.[10] However, if the stones are too large to be extracted through the track, or if one cannot wait 5–6 weeks for the track to mature, then endoscopic sphincterotomy is a very suitable alternative. The presence of the T-tube does not interfere with the sphincterotomy, but it may need to be withdrawn to allow gall-stones to be trapped in the stone basket and removed from the bile duct.

Although the majority of patients referred for endoscopic removal of gall-stones have undergone previous cholecystectomy, there is an increasing trend to consider elderly or medically unfit patients for this procedure if they present with pain and jaundice, even though they have a gall bladder in situ. If the primary problem arises from the bile duct, it would seem reasonable to remove the calculi endoscopically and then either proceed to elective cholecystectomy at a later date, or even decide to leave the gall bladder in situ if the patient is considered unfit for surgery.

Gross obesity which might preclude surgery, presents no problem to the endoscopist, other than physically getting the patient on and off the x-ray table.

The presence of acute cholangitis with or without jaundice used to be regarded as a relative contra-indication to ERCP but this is no longer so. Experience has shown that as soon as the calculi are removed following sphincterotomy, the cholangitis settles very rapidly. Endoscopic sphincterotomy is a particularly safe and effective method of dealing acutely with these extremely ill patients.

Rather like acute cholangitis, the presence of pancreatitis used to be regarded as a contra-indication to ERCP and endoscopic sphincterotomy. European experience has lead us to realize that ERCP may not be so dangerous in the acute phase of pancreatitis as was once thought and the most experienced endoscopists are now happy to perform endoscopic sphincterotomy during the acute phase of gall-stone pancreatitis,[15] particularly if the condition is relapsing or fails to settle with conservative management.

Contra-indications

There are remarkably few contra-indications to endoscopic sphincterotomy and, as already mentioned, age, obesity and associated medical illness are all factors that make the procedure preferable to surgery.

Some anatomical situations make endoscopic sphincterotomy very difficult, if not impossible, but are not actually contra-indications. The presence of a periampullary diverticulum with a papilla inside may prevent cannulation and sphincterotomy, as may a Billroth II partial gastrectomy. It may be possible to pass an endoscope up the afferent loop but due to the inverted approach, sphincterotomy is almost impossible.

The patient who is carrying the hepatitis B antigen is a risk to the clinician and potentially to other patients examined with the same equipment, although with careful attention to detail, avoiding blood contamination and cleaning up meticulously afterwards, such patients can be dealt with safely.

One of the few conditions that make endoscopic sphincterotomy dangerous, is a coagulation defect. As bleeding from the sphincterotomy site is one of the more common, but totally unpredictable, complications of the procedure, the patient must have normal clotting. If the coagulation defect cannot be corrected, then surgery, where direct control of bleeding sites can be more easily obtained, is preferable. In certain situations, if the risks of surgery are greater than endoscopic sphincterotomy, the procedure can be performed with fresh frozen plasma, platelet transfusion or factor concentrates immediately available if needed.

The known presence of extremely large calculi, over 3 cm, make endoscopic sphincterotomy unlikely to succeed and direct removal through a very large sphincterotomy of that size may be hazardous. However, if an adequate sphincterotomy of up to 2 cm in length is performed, together with attempts at reducing the gall-stone size using chemical dissolution therapy (Chapter 5), then large stones can sometimes be extracted successfully.

RESULTS

The results of a personal series of 256 patients with common bile duct calculi referred for endoscopic sphincterotomy at The London Hospital between 1976 and 1983, are shown in Table 8.1. The age range of these patients was 18–96 years with a mean of 62 years. A sphincterotomy was performed successfully in 241 patients (94%). Of the 15 patients (6%) in whom sphincterotomy failed, the papilla was inaccessible inside a diverticulum in 10, three patients had a previous Polya gastrectomy and in two the papilla was not located. The 241 patients in whom a sphincterotomy was performed successfully had a total of 470 common bile duct calculi, and successful clearance of the bile duct calculi was achieved in 217 patients (90%). There was therefore an overall success rate in removing common bile duct calculi in all the patients in this series of 85%.

In the 24 patients in whom the bile duct calculi could not be extracted

Table 8.1

Endoscopic sphincterotomy and gall-stone removal at
The London Hospital, 1976–83.

Total number of patients	256
Sphincterotomy successful	241/256 (94%)
Calculi extracted successfully	217/241 (90%)
Overall success rate	217/256 (85%)

completely, the reason for failure in all but three was the large size of the calculi. Twenty-one of these patients had calculi measuring 1.5 cm or more. The other three patients had smaller calculi above a low bile duct stricture which prevented their removal through the sphincterotomy orifice.

Complications

The various complications encountered in the 241 patients who underwent a successful endoscopic sphincterotomy are listed in Table 8.2. There were 23 patients (9.5%) who suffered complications of the procedure, in nine patients (3.7%) surgery was necessary to deal with these complications. To date, there has been no mortality following endoscopic sphincterotomy nor in the post-operative period following surgery for the complications.

Table 8.2

Complications of endoscopic sphincterotomy[a] and gall-stone removal at The London Hospital, 1976–83.

	Patients		Surgery necessary		Deaths
Type of complication	No.	%	No.	%	No.
Bleeding (needing transfusion)	7	2.9	3	1.2	0
Cholangitis	6	2.5	2	0.8	0
Cholecystitis	2	0.8	2	0.8	0
Pancreatitis	4	1.7	0	0.0	0
Stone basket impaction	3	1.2	2	0.8	0
Gall-stone ileus	1	0.4	0	0.0	0
Retroperiotoneal perforation	0	0.0	0	0.0	0
TOTAL	23	9.5	9	3.7	0

[a]Number of patients undergoing sphincterotomy = 241.

The commonest complication encountered after endoscopic sphinctero-tomy is bleeding from the sphincterotomy site. It is not uncommon to find a little initial bleeding from the edge of the sphincterotomy but occasionally unpredictably severe bleeding can occur, necessitating transfusion and even surgery, if the bleeding does not subside. Invariably such severe bleeding is arterial and arises from a small branch of the superior pancreatico-duodenal artery, which has a variable position, being 0.5–3 cms above the papilla of Vater. In view of this inconsistant relationship of the artery to the papilla, severe bleeding can occur even after small-sized sphincterotomies and is totally unpredictable. If the bleeding does not stop with transfusion, most patients will be managed by simple surgical oversewing of the top of the sphincterotomy but occasionally severe bleeding continues and more radical measures, such as Whipple's pancreatectomy, may have to be considered.

Although it is not uncommon for some patients to experience transitory abdominal pain for 24 hours following the procedure, a true attack of pancreatitis is remarkably uncommon. The pancreatitis probably relates to the diathermy technique used to create the sphincterotomy so close to the pancreatic duct orifice. It is of vital importance, therefore, to make sure that the sphincterotome is completely in the bile duct before starting to apply diathermy current.

Cholangitis following sphincterotomy is invariably caused by large gall-stones impacting at the lower end of the bile duct if they have been left to pass spontaneously. In recent years, the technique of inserting a drainage catheter high in the bile duct and re-routing it through the nose, once the endoscope has been withdrawn, has reduced this sort of complication considerably by providing free drainage while large gall-stones are passing spontaneously. This technique will be discussed later in this chapter. In this series of patients, there were also two episodes of acute cholecystitis within a week of endoscopic sphincterotomy and gall-stone removal in patients who still had their gall-bladder intact. It is unclear whether this was incidental or related to the manipulation within the bile duct.

Impaction of the stone basket usually only occurs when large gall-stones are being extracted and the sphincterotomy is not large enough to allow removal into the duodenum. Sometimes the stone basket and stone will become disimpacted and pass spontaneously into the duodenum after a few days. If this does not happen spontaneously, surgery will be necessary to remove the basket and calculus.

Occasionally, after very large stones have been removed or passed spontaneously from the bile duct into the duodenum, gall-stone ileus can occur. This happened in one patient in this series but settled with conserva-tive measures. Although there are no cases of retroperitoneal perforation in the current series, this occasionally occurs and usually follows an attempt to create a very large sphincterotomy in order to deal with large gall-stones. Such a complication should be noticed immediately, as contrast is seen to leave the bile duct and enter a cavity outside the margins of the duodenum on x-ray screening. Such patients should be managed conservatively initially with nil by mouth, intravenous fluids, and antibiotic cover. Most patients settle on this regime and will not need surgical exploration.

Although there has been no mortality in this particular series, experience from other centres has shown that mortality is usually associated with severe bleeding or sepsis in those patients who would be considered extremely high risk patients for surgery. Very occasionally, severe exsanguinating bleeding can occur in the young and fit patient. This sort of complication is totally unpredictable and whereas it might be regarded as an acceptable risk in the elderly and medically unfit, it would not be regarded as acceptable in the very young.

As the technique is still in its infancy, reports as to long-term complications have still to emerge. There are anecdotal reports of sphincterotomy re-stenosis and recurrent cholangitis in occasional patients with no evidence of recurrent gall-stones. There does not appear to be any reason to expect significant long-term complications to emerge.

Other centres' results and complications

Results from other centres with considerable experience in this technique show a success rate of performing sphincterotomy in about 96% of patients, and successful gall-stone extraction in 92% of patients after sphincterotomy, giving an overall success rate of gall-stone extraction in 89% of patients.[16] Reported complication rates from various series are very similar to those stated in Table 8.2 and there is a small mortality rate which is usually under 1% in experienced hands.[17,18] There is no doubt that greater experience of the individual endoscopist leads to better results, as a multi-centre study has recently shown.[17] In this review of the British experience of endoscopic sphincterotomy, it was apparent that centres in which there was limited experience of the technique, had less success in performing sphincterotomy and removing gall-stones. Although their complication rate was similar to those with more experience, their mortality rate was higher.

PROBLEM AREAS

Large calculi

Many of the cases of failed gall-stone extraction, and complications such as cholangitis and stone impaction, relate to the presence of very large calculi that cannot be removed actively or fail to pass spontaneously through a normal-sized endoscopic sphincterotomy. In general, most calculi of 1.5 cm diameter and under present little problem, but calculi over 1.5 cm, particularly 2–3 cm diameter, can be extremely difficult to remove. As already mentioned, very large sphincterotomies carry the additional risk of bleeding and retroduodenal perforation. A technique has been developed, which we and other centres now use routinely in the presence of large stones. After the endoscopic sphincterotomy has been performed, and if the stones are too large to remove on that occasion, a radiological guide-wire is passed down the channel of the endoscope and inserted high into the bile duct above the gall-stone. A long pig-tail drainage catheter, with multiple side holes at its distal end, is passed over this guide-wire. This is positioned high in the bile duct (Fig. 8.7) and the endoscope is then removed, leaving the drainage catheter in situ (Fig. 8.8). This catheter is then re-routed from the mouth through the nose and is left draining freely into a bag.[19] This will minimize the risk of jaundice and cholangitis while, it is hoped, large gall-stones are passing spontaneously. There are two additional advantages to this technique. First, repeated tube cholangiograms can be performed down the catheter to monitor the progress of gall-stone passage, and as soon as the bile duct is clear of stones the catheter can be removed without the need for a second ERCP. Secondly, if on repeat cholangiography the gall-stones show no sign of passing spontaneously, then a continuous infusion of mono-ctanoin can be administered via the nasobiliary catheter.[20] In our experience, after 7–10 days of mono-octanoin infusion at a rate of 1–5 ml/hour, gall-stone size is often reduced markedly. The calculi often become softened and friable, and it is then relatively easy to fragment them using a stone basket at the time of a second ERCP when the bile duct can be cleared successfully of stones.

Difficult access to the papilla of Vater

There are two conditions particularly that cause problems in locating the papilla of Vater and performing a sphincterotomy. After a Billroth II partial gastrectomy, performing an ERCP via the afferent loop is in itself technically difficult. To be able to create an adequate endoscopic sphincterotomy and extract gall-stones is even more difficult, and usually impossible in view of the anatomical arrangements.

Where the papilla of Vater is in relationship to a periampullary diverticulum, there may also be difficulties in performing an ERCP and proceeding to sphincterotomy. The papilla may be on the edge or even inside the diverticulum and the direction of the bile duct around the diverticulum makes manipulation difficult. In a recent study, we have found that there is an increased incidence of peri-ampullary diverticula not just in the elderly, but also in patients with common bile duct calculi.[21] The course of the lower bile duct around a diverticulum probably leads to failure of spontaneous gall-stone passage and encourages gall-stone growth in the bile duct itself. If

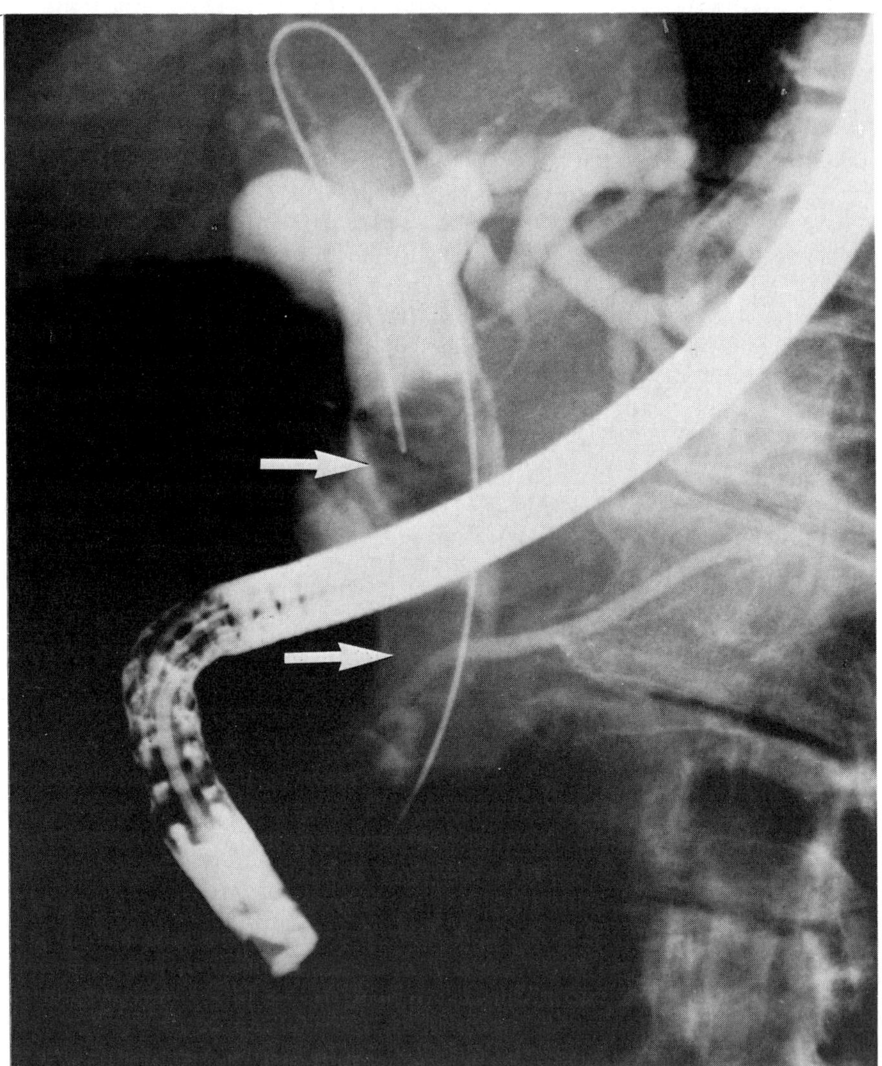

Fig. 8.7 An ERCP showing two large stones (arrows) in the bile duct after sphincterotomy. A guide-wire has been looped high in the bile duct, over which a pig-tail biliary drainage catheter will be passed before the endoscope is removed.

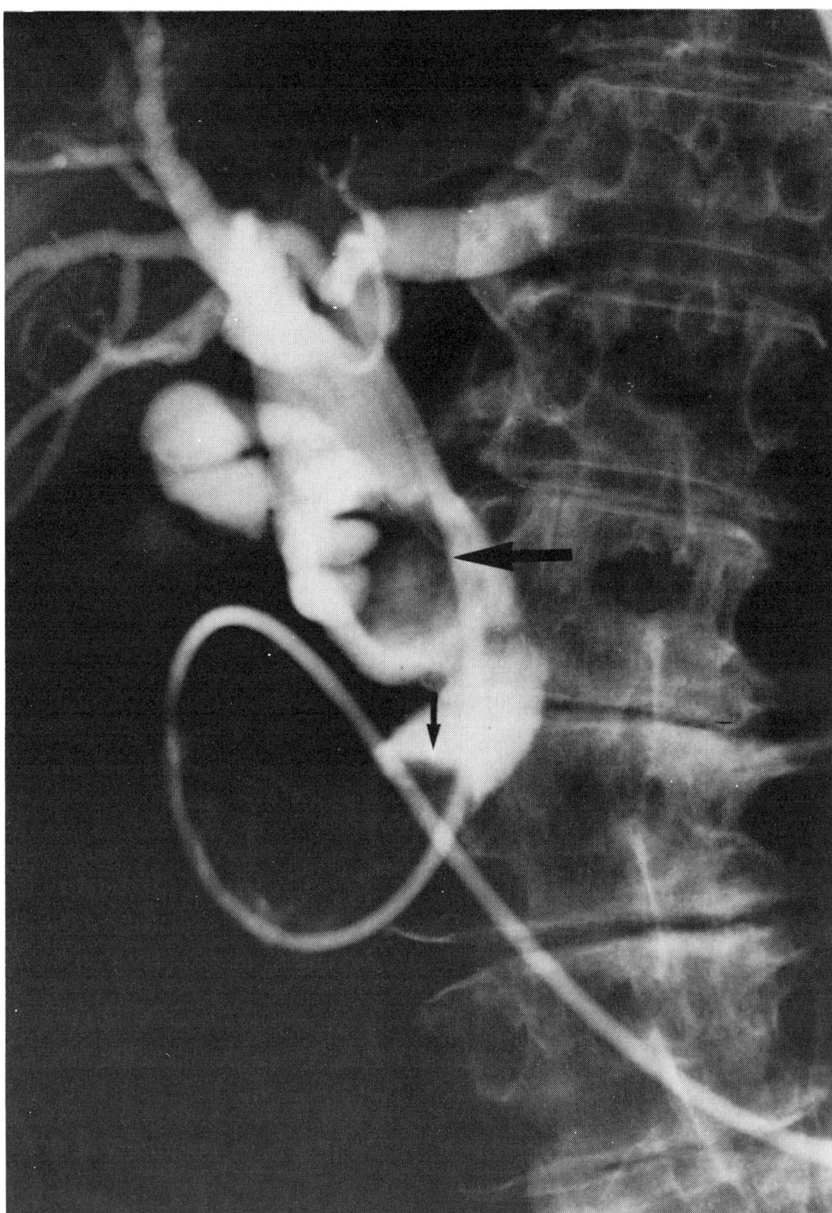

Fig. 8.8 The nasobiliary catheter in situ in the bile duct some days later. The lower stone has almost passed into the duodenum (small arrow); the large calculus can still be seen in the mid bile duct (large arrow).

the papilla is inside the diverticulum and inaccessible to endoscopic cannulation, a combined transhepatic and endoscopic technique can be used in order to remove the calculi non-operatively.[21] Initially, a transhepatic cholangiogram is performed and a catheter inserted into the biliary tree percutaneously. A guide-wire is then inserted down this catheter and passed out of the bile duct into the lumen of the duodenum. This inevitably brings the papilla into view within the lumen of the duodenum. If necessary, a Gruntzig balloon catheter can be passed transhepatically and the papillary orifice dilated under simultaneous, direct endoscopic vision. After this, it is usually a relatively simple matter to perform a straightforward endoscopic sphincterotomy and proceed to extract the common bile duct calculi (Figs 8.9, 8.10).

Patients with intact gall bladders

When first introduced, endoscopic sphincterotomy was restricted to patients who had already undergone cholecystectomy. There are now increasing numbers of patients referred for endoscopic sphincterotomy with their gall bladders still in situ. The overall incidence of such patients in our series was 19%, but in the last year 50% of patients referred had not had a previous cholecystectomy. This same trend has been reported by other authors, who followed 71 elderly patients with intact gall bladders after endoscopic sphincterotomy.[22] Two patients needed emergency cholecystectomy for cholecystitis following the procedure and 11 proceeded to elective cholecystectomy. Of the 48 patients who left hospital with their gall bladders in situ, only five (10.4%) needed cholecystectomy for biliary pain within a two-year follow-up period. In a large series from France, 234 patients with gall bladders in situ were treated. Immediate complications occurred in 7% and mortality was 1.5%.[23] Late complications occurred in 16 patients (12%), of which the most common was cholecystitis.[6]

There is still controversy as to whether elderly but fit patients who have not had previous surgery, should have an initial endoscopic sphincterotomy and later an elective cholecystectomy, or whather they should have both the bile duct and gall bladder dealt with at one operation.[24] At present, controlled trials are in progress to try to answer this question. In the patients who are unfit for surgery it would seem reasonable to leave them with their gall bladders in situ following endoscopic sphincterotomy and pursue an expectant policy.

SUMMARY

Endoscopic sphincterotomy and gall-stone removal offers a relatively safe and effective way of removing common bile duct calculi, and would appear

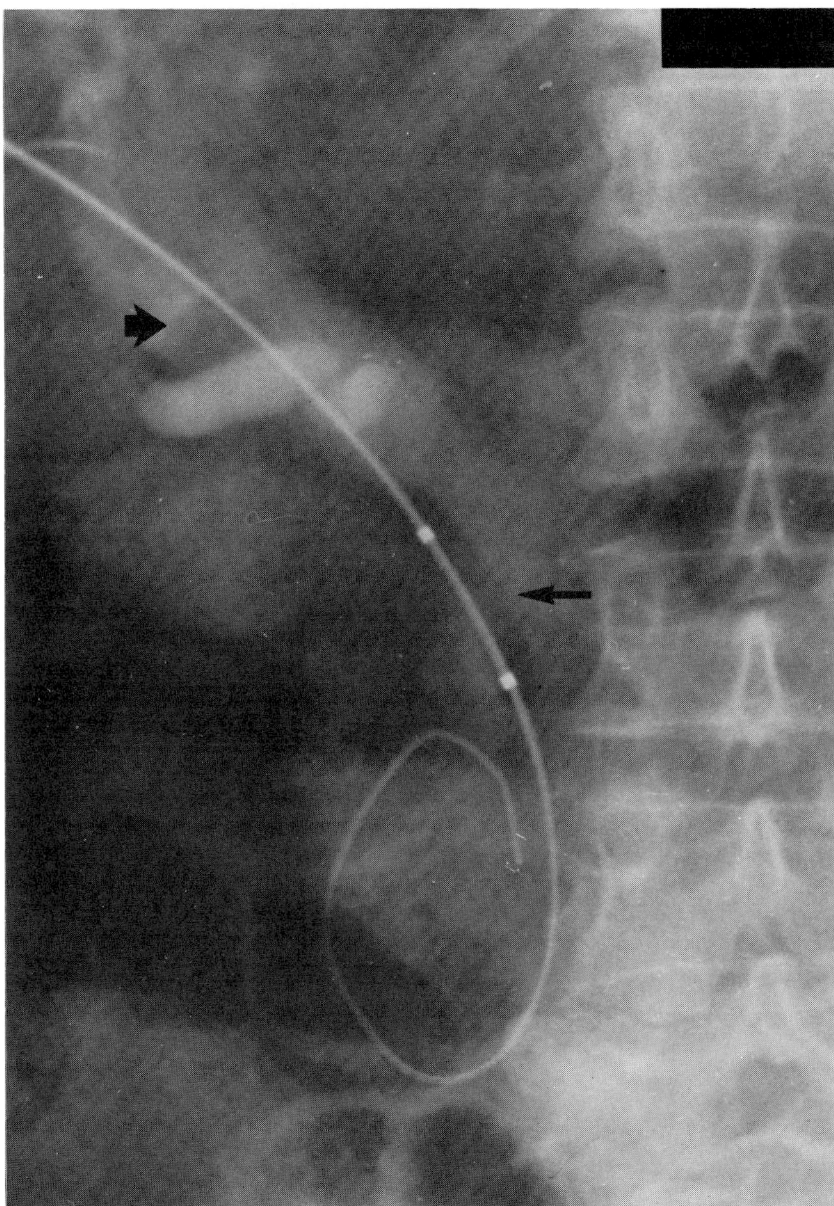

Fig. 8.9   In this x-ray the gall-stone can be seen (large arrow) in a dilated bile duct. A Gruntzig catheter has been passed over a transhepatic biliary guide-wire and the inflated balloon (small arrow) used to dilate the papilla of Vater to facilitate the endoscopic sphincterotomy.

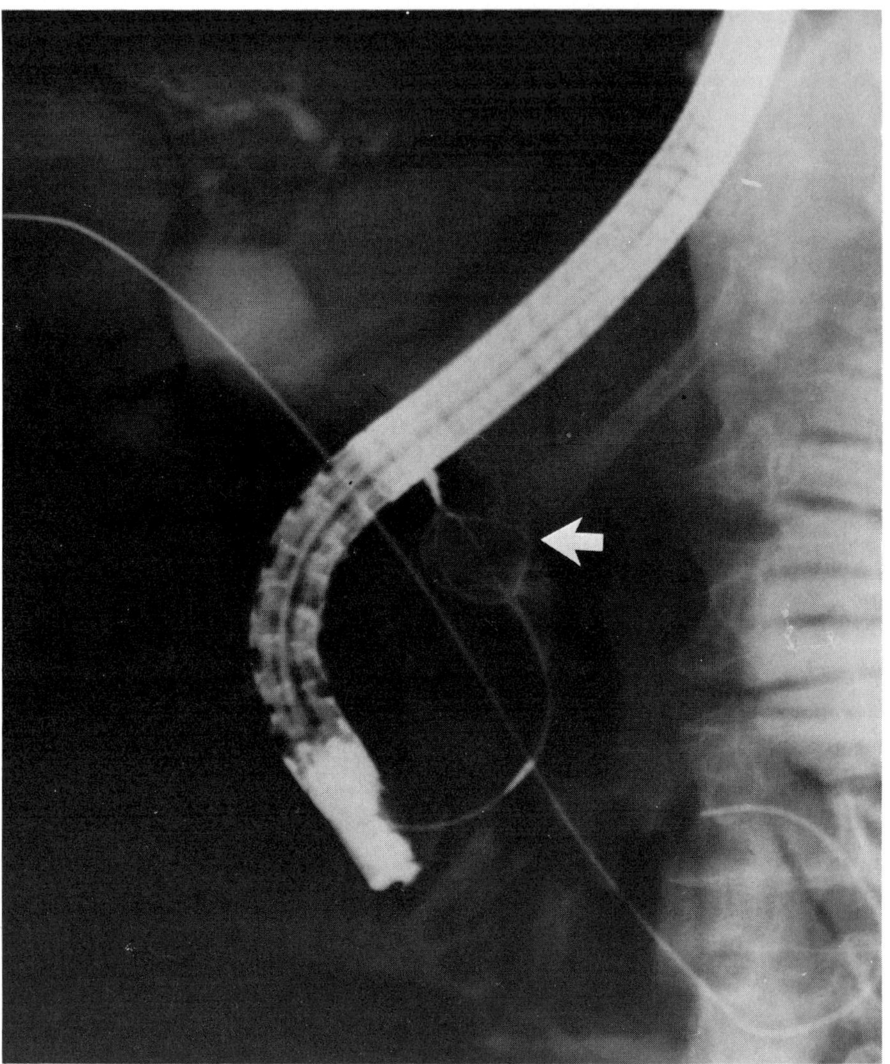

Fig. 8.10   After sphincterotomy has been performed the calculus has been trapped successfully in a stone basket (arrow) and can be removed.

to be preferable to surgery in the patient who has already undergone previous cholecystectomy, particularly in the elderly and medically unfit. The technique can also avoid the need for emergency surgery in the sick patients with acute cholangitis or pancreatitis due to an impacted gall-stone. There is an increasing trend to manage patients who have not had previous biliary surgery and who present with obstructive jaundice due to gall-stones, with endoscopic sphincterotomy. Having removed the common bile duct calculi endoscopically, an elective cholecystectomy can be performed at a later date if necessary.

REFRENCES

1. Classen M, Safrany L. Endoscopic papillotomy and removal of gallstones. Brit Med J 4: 371–374, 1975.
2. Koch H, Classen M, Schaffner O et al. Endoscopic papillotomy. Experimental studies and initial clinical experience. Scand J Gastroenterol 10: 441–444, 1975.
3. Sloof M, Baker R, Lavelle M et al. What is involved in endoscopic sphincterotomy for gallstones? Brit J Surg 67: 18–21, 1980.
4. Mazzeo RJ, Jordan FT, Strasius SR. Endoscopic papillotomy for recurrent common bile duct stones and papillary stenosis. A community hospital experience. Arch Surg 118: 693–695, 1983.
5. McSherry CK, Glenn F. The incidence and causes of death following for non-malignant biliary tract disease. Ann Surg 191: 271–275, 1980.
6. Glenn F. Trends in surgical treatment of calculous disease of the biliary tract. Surg Gynecol Obstet 140: 877–844, 1975.
7. Girard RM, Legros G. Retained and recurrent bile duct stones. Surgical or non-surgical removal? Ann Surg 193: 150–154, 1981.
8. Sphon K, Fux HD, Mehnert U et al. Cholecystektomie und choledochotomie — taktik and techniken. Langenbecks Arch Chir 334: 249, 1973.
9. Thompson JE, Tompkins RK, Longmire WP Jr. Factors in management of acute cholangitis. Ann Surg 195: 137–145, 1982.
10. Allen B, Shapiro H, Way LW. Management of recurrent and residual common duct stones. Am J Surg 142: 41–47, 1981.
11. Koch H, Rosch W, Schaffner O et al. Endoscopic papillotomy. Gastroenterology 73: 1393–1396, 1977.
12. Safrany L. Endoscopic treatment of biliary tract disease. Lancet ii: 983–985, 1978.
13. Mee AS, Vallon AG, Croker JR et al. Non-operative removal of bile duct stones by duodenoscopic sphincterotomy in the elderly. Brit Med J 283: 521–523, 1981.
14. Burhenne HJ. Non-operative removal of bilary tract stones: extraction through post-operative drainage tract. Development of digestive diseases. Philadelphia, Lee & Febiger, pp. 119–126, 1979.
15. Safrany L, Cotton PB. A preliminary report. Urgent duodenoscopic sphincterotomy for acute gallstone pancreatitis. Surgery 89: 424–428, 1981.
16. Cotton PB. Non-operative removal of bile duct stones by duodenoscopic sphincterotomy. Brit J Surg 67: 1–5, 1980.
17. Cotton PB, Vallon AG. British experience with duodenoscopic sphincterotomy for removal of bile duct stones. Brit J Surg 68: 373–375, 1981.
18. Ghazi A, McSherry CK. Endoscopic retrograde cholangiopancreatography and sphincterotomy. Ann Surg 199: 21–27, 1984.
19. Cotton PB, Burney PGJ, Mason RR. Transnasal bile duct catheterisation after endoscopic sphincterotomy. Gut 20: 285–287, 1979.

20. Venu RP, Geenen JE, Toouli J et al. Gallstone dissolution using mono-octanoin infusion through an endoscopically placed nasobiliary catheter. Am J Gastroenterol 77: 227–230, 1982.
21. Hatfield ARW, Murray AS, Lennard-Jones JE. Periampullary diverticula and common duct calculi: a combined transhepatic and endoscopic technique for difficult cases. Gut 23: 889, 1982.
22. Cotton PB, Vallon AG. Duodenoscopic sphincteroromy for removal of bile duct stones in patients with gallbladders. Surgery 91: 628–630, 1982.
23. Escourrou J, Cordova JA, Lazorthes F et al. Early and late complications after endoscopic sphincterotomy for biliary lithiasis with and without the gall bladder 'in situ'. Gut 5: 598–602, 1984.
24. Cotton PB. Endoscopic management of bile duct stones; (apples and oranges). Gut 25: 587–597, 1984.

9

Surgical Management of Recurrent Common Duct Stones

Nicolas J. Lygidakis

Biliary lithiasis has challenged the medical profession for thousands of years. However, surgical intervention for cure or for relief was not introduced until the nineteenth century.[1] Today, despite dramatic advances in diagnostic and therapeutic techniques, biliary lithiasis continues to be a major clinical problem.

It is estimated that 12 million women and 4 million men in the U.S.A. alone have gall-stones, and each year 800,000 new cases will appear.[2] Apart from any early morbidity or mortality associated with the initial operation, there is a late morbidity, largely due to retained or recurrent stones and biliary strictures. Between 500,000 and 800,000 patients undergo surgery, and of these approximately 8000 will be re-operations.[3,4]

Recurrent choledocholithiasis, despite progress in modern pre- and intra-operative technology, continues to be a challenge for the surgeon. Apart from further discomfort to the patient and embarrassment to the surgeon, re-exploration of the common bile duct is associated with two additional distressing features: (1) an operative mortality twice that of the primary choledochotomy, and four times that of uncomplicated cholecystectomy,[5] and (2) a higher incidence of residual or retained common bile duct calculi — 10% — which, after a third or fourth subsequent common bile duct re-exploration, may well be much higher.[6]

Consequently, the author believes that in order to appreciate objectively what each therapeutic approach can offer, it is necessary to outline aspects of the aetiology, and particularly the pathogenesis, of recurrent choledocholithiasis. Despite routine use of intra-operative cholangiography with or without the use of choledochoscopy, there remains a proportion of patients — varying from 2 to 10% — who, despite meticulous clearance of all stones from their bile ducts, develop recurrent bile duct calculi at various time intervals after their initial surgery.[7-15] Complete eradication of calculous material from the biliary ductal system in all patients with choledocholithiasis remains a desired, but still unaccomplished, achievement of modern medicine.

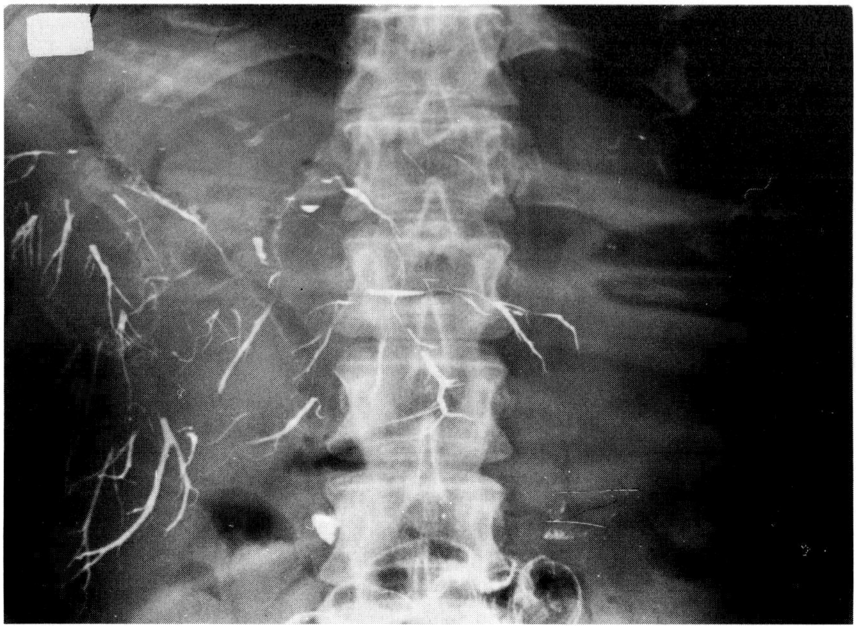

Fig. 9.1 Delayed emptying of biliary tree in a patient with longstanding choledocholithiasis. Barium is retained in the intrahepatic bile ducts for one week.

It has been demonstrated in patients of advanced age with a long history of symptoms of biliary lithiasis, that biliary stasis is a prominent feature of their disease, and this is reflected in their inability to empty the biliary system adequately[14] (Figs 9.1 and 9.2). In addition, it has been shown that in such patients there is a high incidence of pathological change of both liver and biliary tree histology (Figs 9.3 and 9.4), and that this is associated with a high incidence of bile infection, primary common bile duct stones, and common bile duct dilatation.[15-19] Furthermore, it has been shown that the above findings persist long after the relief of the obstruction, but that they gradually return to normal provided a free and unimpeded flow of bile from the liver to the duodenum is established.[20,21] It is interesting that in a series of patients, all of whom underwent surgery for recurrent choledocholithiasis, the above-mentioned features were seen frequently.[22] It has been shown clearly in these patients that there is a close correlation between the incidence of bile infection and primary common bile duct stones.[22] It seems likely that any type of management, and particularly surgical management, should necessarily take these features into consideration.

In a recent prospective randomized study,[20] a series of patients presenting for treatment of recurrent choledocholithiasis, with the above-mentioned

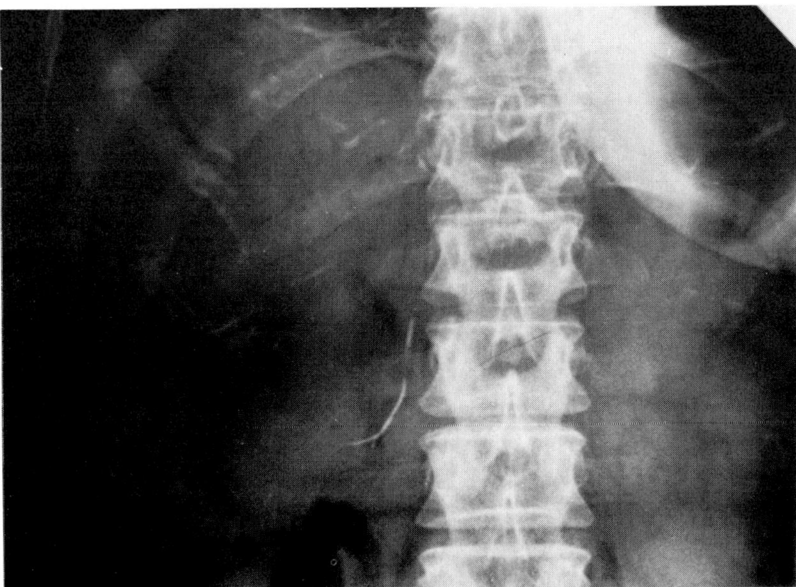

Fig. 9.2   Another patient with longstanding choledocholithiasis. Barium is retained in the intrahepatic bile ducts one month after its insertion.

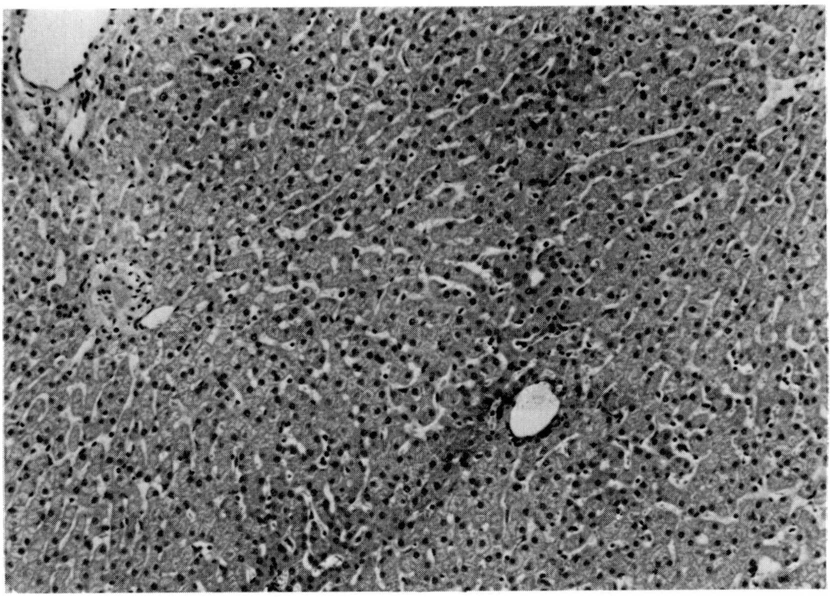

Fig. 9.3   Liver histology of a patient with longstanding choledocholithiasis. Note the newly formed intrahepatic bile ducts with features of periportal fibrosis.

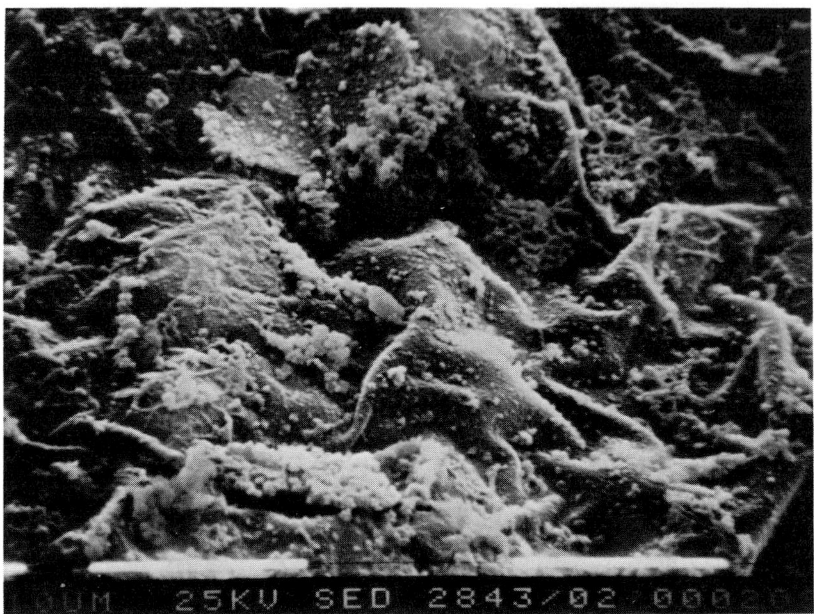

Fig. 9.4 Scanning electron micrograph of a patient with a dilated biliary tree. There is complete destruction of the linear epithelium of the common bile duct, which has a crater-like appearance.

operative and clinical characteristics, were assessed to determine the effects of a supplementary procedure after choledochotomy and stone extraction. Patients either underwent closure of the common bile duct with T-tube drainage or choledochoduodenostomy. Results showed that only after choledochoduodenostomy was the establishment of free bile flow to the duodenum accomplished, and the overall incidence of recurrent choledocholithiasis was almost entirely eliminated. In contrast, when choledochotomy and stone extraction were supplemented by T-tube drainage alone there was a high incidence of recurrent choledocholithiasis, presumably due to the persistence of biliary stasis. The above results highlight the fact that only when biliary stasis is eliminated is recurrent choledocholithiasis abolished, and that this can be achieved only through a drainage procedure supplementary to choledochotomy.

It is interesting that in the above series of patients intra-operative cholangiography was routine, and that all patients with recurrent choledocholithiasis underwent further surgery[5] 5–9 years after initial surgery. The same findings were reported in another study,[21] emphasizing that in the presence of biliary stasis, which is frequently seen in patients presenting for treatment of recurrent choledocholithiasis, the surgeon must not only clear the bile ducts of stones, but must also abolish biliary stasis. Another feature is the higher mortality and earlier morbidity rate associated with choledochotomy and T-tube drainage than is seen after choledochotomy supplemented by choledochoduodenostomy.[20] Similarly, in subsequent studies[22,23] where T-tube drainage was compared to choledochoduodenostomy in a series of patients with infected bile, it was shown that internal drainage — choledochoduodenostomy — was associated with far better results in terms of mortality and early morbidity than T-tube drainage; this was more obvious in cases of acute septic cholangitis.

The above findings are important when dealing with patients with recurrent choledocholithiasis in whom it is known that there is a high incidence of bile infection, biliary tree dilatation, advanced pathological changes of the liver and biliary ductal apparatus, and primary common bile duct stones.[24]

We should remember that in treating recurrent choledocholithiasis, biliary calculi are not the entire disease but merely the presenting symptom. This holds true for a great proportion of patients seen with recurrent choledocholithiasis. Indeed, it would appear likely that such patients may well harbour primary gall-stones within their dilated bile ducts, and that recurrent stones may appear even after the most precise clearance of the duct. Thus, it seems reasonable when dealing with patients with recurrent choledocholithiasis to consider carefully the various indications for a supplementary drainage procedure, in addition to choledochotomy, in order to eliminate the disease completely.

Common drainage procedures used after choledochotomy are choledochoduodenostomy (Fig. 9.5), hepaticojejunostomy (Fig. 9.6), and sphincteroplasty (Fig. 9.7).[25-30] Choledochoduodenostomy has many advantages when compared to sphincteroplasty. It adds little to the operative time, and is a safe and simple procedure which, when used with proper indications, is associated with very satisfactory results.[25-28] In contrast, operative mortality and morbidity after sphincteroplasty is higher, and the overall incidence of complications related to the procedure (i.e. post-operative pancreatitis), rather than complications of surgery in general, are more common than after choledochoduodenostomy. Although excellent results have been reported by some after sphincteroplasty,[29,30] others have reported less promising results.[31]

In a recent study,[31] where both choledochoduodenostomy and sphincteroplasty were carried out prospectively in a randomly selected series of patients with recurrent choledocholithiasis, it was shown that choledochoduodenostomy was associated with better results than sphincteroplasty. Not only was the mortality and early morbidity lower, but also the late morbidity

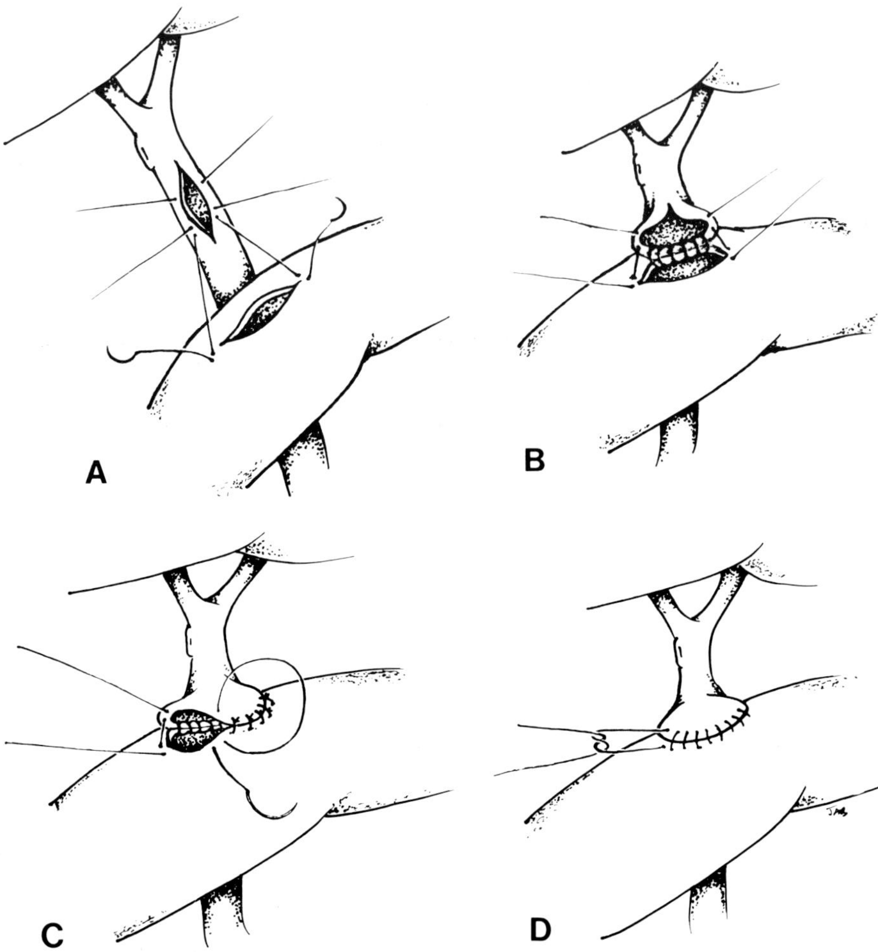

Fig. 9.5 (A–D) Choledochoduodenostomy side-to-side anastomosis between the common bile duct and the duodenum.

and overall re-operation rate was markedly reduced after choledochoduode-nostomy.[31] These findings were supported by another study[14] in which barium meal follow-through studies were performed through the constructed choledochoduodenostomy. The progress of pathological changes on the liver and biliary tree histology post-operatively was reflected by the radiological findings. Liver and common bile duct biopsies were taken in another series of patients with longstanding extrahepatic biliary obstruction who underwent choledochoduodenostomy after choledochotomy and stone extraction. Twenty days post-operatively, barium meal follow-through

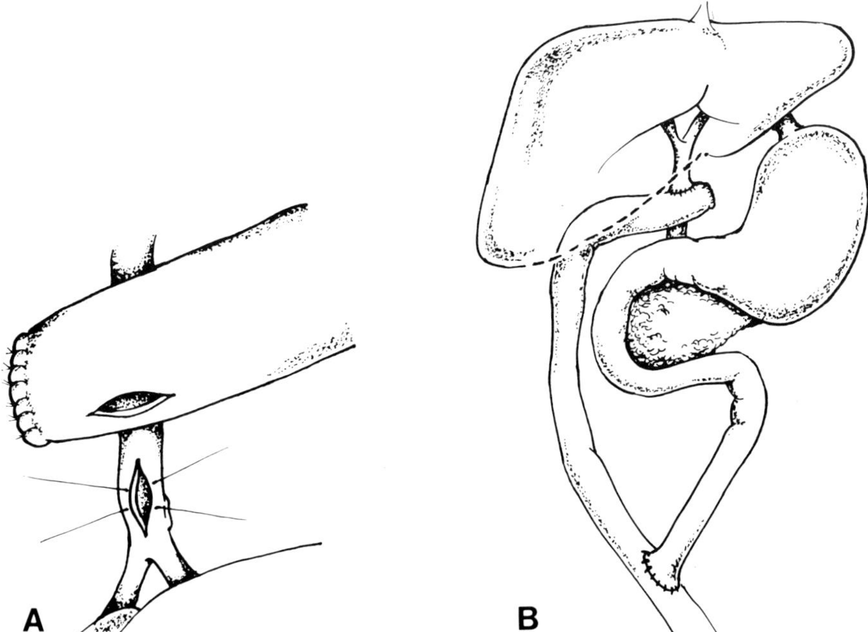

Fig. 9.6   (A–B) Hepaticojejunostomy end-to-side anastomosis between the hepatic duct and a Roux-en-Y isolated jejunal loop.

studies were carried out and the filling and emptying time of the entire intra- and extrahepatic biliary tree, and more precisely its appearance and visualization, were assessed carefully, and related to our histological findings.

It has been shown clearly that the biliary tree pathology persists for many years after the relief of extrahepatic biliary obstruction, and that biliary stasis is a prominent feature which, if left untreated, would certainly lead to formation of further biliary calculi. That the above findings were seen to return towards normal after choledochoduodenostomy weighs heavily in favour of this procedure in re-establishing normal histology of the liver and biliary tree, and in eliminating biliary stasis and the incidence of recurrent choledocholithiasis.

On the other hand, secondary stenosis or inadequate drainage was significantly more frequent following sphincteroplasty than after choledochoduodenostomy which, although reported, occurs seldom and only when the procedure is carried out on a narrow common bile duct. Nevertheless, there are some who oppose the use of the above biliary drainage procedures on the grounds that both are associated with an increased late morbidity due to cholangitis; this is often the consequence of reflux of duodenal contents

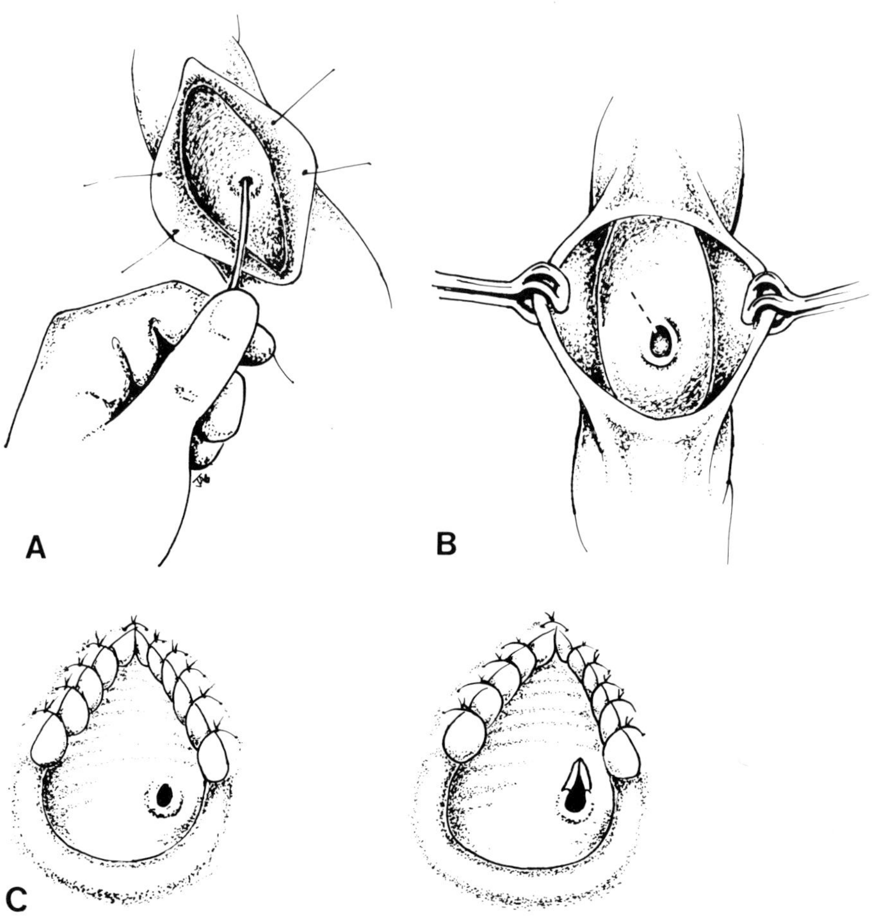

Fig. 9.7 (A–C) Sphincteroplasty. Opening of the duodenum. Identification of the papilla and large sphincteroplasty.

into the distal bile duct after sphincteroplasty, or the "sump" syndrome, caused by debris remaining or accumulating within the intrapancreatic portion of bile duct, after choledochoduodenostomy.

Although the author has performed choledochojejunostomy in a number of patients, the procedure can not be recommended as there is no proof of its superiority in the management of patients with recurrent choledocholithiasis. However, there has been satisfactory experience in carrying out side-to-side choledochoduodenostomy in a larger series of patients with recurrent choledocholithiasis, and in whom indications and techniques similar to those advocated by others[25–28] were used[31] (Table 9.1). The results were graded

Table 9.1

Mortality and morbidity rates in 564 patients who underwent biliary drainage by use of different procedures supplementary to choledochotomy.

Procedure	No. of patients	Deaths	Wound infection	Respiratory infections	DVT	Pulmonary embolism	Total percentage of complications
Primary choledochoduodenostomy	250	—	10	1	—	—	4.4
Choledochoduodenostomy after choledochotomy	132	4	20	3	4	3	22.7
Primary sphincteroplasty	19	—	1	1	—	—	10.5
Sphincteroplasty after choledochotomy	96	3	14	2	4	—	20.8
Choledochojejunostomy after choledochotomy or after choledochotomy and T-tube drainage	67	1	14	3	2	2	36.2
TOTAL	564	8	59	10	10	5	

and the clinical response assessed in relation to the progress of various liver function tests at intervals after the above procedures. There was a far better outcome and a lower incidence of various post-operative sequelae after choledochoduodenostomy than after either sphincteroplasty or choledocho-jejunostomy (Table 9.2). Additionally, there were two patients who, despite having an open and patent stoma after sphincteroplasty, developed marked fibrosis at the margins of the stoma with an advanced peristomal inflammation and proximal hold-up of debris, with consequent dilatation of the biliary tree and frequent attacks of cholangitis.

Today, the advent of endoscopic papillotomy allows successful removal of residual common bile duct stones in a proportion of patients presenting with recurrent choledocholithiasis. This is not a handicap to surgical management of the above disease, but an alternative which can be of value in a number of selected cases. However, in a recent report,[32] there was an 11% overall failure rate to remove the stones in a series of 134 patients in whom endoscopic papillotomy was carried out. Safrany[33] reported similar results. In addition, complications occurred in 10 out of 134 patients, three of whom required emergency surgery, and of those three, one died. A 38% failure rate in the removal of stones was noted when the stone was greater than 2 cm.[33] In another series in the United Kingdom,[34] a bed occupancy of 9.5 ($\pm$ 5) days was reported for endoscopic papillotomy, with a clear duct in only 70% of the patients and with a complication rate of 30%. One patient, 37 years old, died as a result of the procedure, and another patient died a year later; this death was also attributed to a complication which might have been avoided if surgery had been carried out initially.

A recently published survey of British centres employing endoscopic sphincterotomy for removal of common bile duct stones has shown that the overall success rate in carrying out the above technique is 76%.[35] Seven deaths — 1% — were recorded from a total number of 679 endoscopic papillotomies, of which only 590 were successful. Overall, early morbidity rate was 8.9%. It is noteworthy that when complications arise after endoscopic papillotomy the majority of them are related to haemorrhage, pancreatitis, and cholangitis, and are associated with a high mortality rate. Indeed, in 58 patients with complications, 11 required an operation within hours or a few days, and seven of those died.[35] Additionally, the precise nature and extent of endoscopic sphincterotomy required to achieve control and long-term results in terms of recurrent or re-stenosis is not yet clearly known.

In contrast, mortality and morbidity after surgery for recurrent choledocholithiasis is less than 2%.[36] In an analysis of six recent series of re-operations for retained or recurrent bile duct stones there was a mortality rate of 1.8% in 498 operations, most of them being in elderly patients.[36] In

Table 9.2

Most recent results in 564 patients who underwent biliary drainage by use of different surgical procedures supplementary to choledochotomy.

Procedure	No. of patients	No. of patients who attended follow-up	Grade I	Grade II	Grade III	Grade IV
Primary choledochoduodenostomy	250	190	162	23	5	—
Choledochoduodenostomy after a previous choledochotomy and T-tube drainage	132	90	79	6	5	—
Primary sphincteroplasty	19	14	9	3	2	—
Sphincteroplasty after choledochotomy T-tube drainage	96	84	63	14	6	3
Choledochojejunostomy after either choledochoduodenostomy or choledochotomy T-tube drainage	67	60	48	6	6	–
TOTAL	564	438	361	52	24	3

another series,[37] 341 patients were reported in whom choledocholithotomy was carried out for retained or recurrent calculi. Of those, 2.1% died, but if patients with cholangitis and pancreatitis were excluded only four (1.2%) died after secondary choledocholithotomy.[37]

Thus, the acceptance of endoscopic papillotomy on the basis of a lower mortality and morbidity rate, in comparison to surgical therapy, appears to be unjustified. However, there is no doubt that the above figures for mortality and morbidity following secondary choledochotomy would definitely be higher if there is surgical interference to the sphincter of Oddi. The majority of deaths are the consequence of acute pancreatitis.[31]

In conclusion, the author believes that in the management of individual patients with recurrent choledocholithiasis, surgery should be considered as an approach of choice, except in the very old and really poor-risk patients for whom endoscopic sphincterotomy might well be indicated. Surgery for retained or recurrent stones in patients with dilated ducts who frequently have a high incidence of pathological changes of the liver and biliary tree, and a high incidence of bile infection, should be supplemented by a drainage procedure which abolishes biliary stasis, and virtually eliminates further recurrence of the disease. From the spectrum of personal experience, and also from the results published in the literature, the author recommends choledochoduodenostomy rather than choledochojejunostomy or sphincteroplasty. Sphincteroplasty should be carried out only in the presence of stones impacted in the ampulla, and choledochojejunostomy should seldom be used except in the presence of duodenal ulceration, when the fashioning of a large choledochoduodenostomy might technically not be feasible.

REFERENCES

1. Bobbs JS. Case of lithotomy of gallbladder. Trans Indiana State Med Soc 18: 68–70, 1868.
2. Small DM. The etiology and pathogenesis of gallstones. Advances in Surgery, Vol 10 (WP Longmire Jr Ed), Chicago, Year Book Medical, pp. 63–85, 1976.
3. Way LW. Retained common duct stones. Surg Clin N Amer 53: 1139–1148, 1973.
4. Safrany L. Duodenoscopic sphincterotomy and gallstone removal. Gastroenterology 72: 338–345, 1977.
5. Kune GA. Current Practice of Biliary Surgery, Boston, Little Brown, 1972.
6. Lygidakis NJ. Early re-operation after surgery for calculous biliary tract disease. Brit J Clin Prac 36: 127–132, 1982.
7. Moss JP, Whelan JG, Dedman TC III et al. Post-operative choledochoscopy through the T-tube tract. Surg Gynecol Obstet 151: 807–811, 1980.
8. Farha GJ, Pearson RN. Transcystic duct operative cholangiography. Personal experience with 500 consecutive cases. Amer J Surg 131: 228–233, 1976.

9. Feliciano DV, Mattox KL, Jordan GL. The value of choledochoscopy in exploration of the common bile duct. Ann Surg. 192: 649–655, 1980.

10. Finnis D, Rowntree T. Choledochoscopy in exploration of the common bile duct. Brit J Surg 64: 661–664, 1977.

11. White TT, Bordley J IV. One per cent incidence of recurrent gallstones six to eight years after manometric cholangiography. Ann Surg 188: 562–569, 1978.

12. Glenn F. Retained calculi within the biliary ductal system. Ann Surg 179: 528–532, 1974.

13. Tondelli P, Gyr J, Stalder GA et al. The biliary tract. Part I: cholecystectomy. Clin Gastroenterol 8: 487–499, 1979.

14. Longmire WP Jr. The diverse causes of biliary obstruction and their remedies. Curr Prob Surg 14: 1–6, 1977.

15. Lygidakis NJ. Surgical approaches to postcholecystectomy choledocholithiasis. Arch Surg 117: 481–489, 1982.

16. Lygidakis NJ. Histologic changes and intrahepatic biliary abnormalities in extrahepatic biliary tract obstruction. Surg Gynecol Obstet 153: 532–539, 1981.

17. Lygidakis NJ. Bile infection: its incidence and significance in biliary lithiasis. Amer J Gastroenterol 77: 210–218, 1982.

18. Lygidakis NJ. Abnormal drainage of the biliary tree after relief of long-standing extrahepatic biliary obstruction. Amer J Surg 146: 318–321, 1983.

19. Lygidakis NJ. The incidence and significance of common bile duct dilatation in biliary calculous diseases. World J Surg 8: 327–334, 1984.

20. Lygidakis NJ. Surgical approaches to recurrent choledocholithiasis: choledochoduodenostomy versus T-tube drainage after choledochotomy. Amer J Surg 145: 636–644, 1983.

21. Saharia PC, Zuidema GD, Cameron JL. Primary common duct stones. Ann Surg 185: 598–604, 1977.

22. Lygidakis NJ. Acute suppurative cholangitis: comparison of internal and external biliary drainage. Am J Surg 143: 304–306, 1982.

23. Lygidakis NJ. Infective complications after choledochotomy. Incidence after T-tube drainage of the common bile duct or after choledochoduodenostomy. J R Coll Surg Edin 27: 233–239, 1982.

24. Lygidakis NJ. Incidence and significance of primary stones of the common bile duct in choledocholithiasis. Surg Gynecol Obstet 158: 434–439, 1983.

25. Schein CJ, Shapiro N, Gliedman ML. Choledochoduodenostomy as an adjunct to choledocholithotomy. Surg Gynecol Obstet 146: 25–29, 1978.

26. Madden SL, Chun SY, Kandalaft S et al. Choledochoduodenostomy: an unjustly maligned surgical procedure. Amer J Surg 119: 45–49, 1970.

27. Lygidakis NJ. Choledochoduodenostomy for calculous biliary tract disease. Brit J Surg 68: 762–768, 1981.

28. Degenshein GA. Choledochoduodenostomy. An 18 year study of 175 consecutive cases. Surgery 76: 319–323, 1974.

29. Jones SA. Sphincteroplasty (not Sphincterotomy) in the treatment of biliary tract disease. Surg Clin N Amer 53: 1123–1129, 1973.

30. Partington PF. Twenty-three years of experience with sphincterotomy and sphincteroplasty for stenosis of the sphincter of Oddi. Surg Gynecol Obstet 145: 161–167, 1977.

31. Lygidakis NJ. A prospective randomized study of recurrent choledocholithiasis. Surg Gynecol Obstet 155: 679–684, 1982.

32. Cotton PB. Non-operative removal of bile duct stones by duodenoscopic sphincterotomy. Brit J Surg 67: 1–9, 1980.
33. Safrany L. Endoscopic treatment of biliary tract diseases. Lancet ii: 983–988, 1978.
34. Sloof M, Baker, Lavelle MI et al. What is involved in endoscopic sphincterotomy for gallstones? Brit J Surg 67: 18–24, 1980.
35. Cotton PB, Vallon AG. British experience with duodenoscopic sphincterotomy for removal of bile duct stones. Brit J Surg 68: 373–379, 1981.
36. Girard RM, Legros G. Retained and recurrent bile duct stones. Surgical or nonsurgical removal? Ann Surg 193: 150–158, 1981.
37. McSherry CK, Glenn F. The incidence and cause of death following surgery for nonmalignant biliary tract disease. Ann Surg 191: 271–278, 1980.

Index